Sleep and Psychiatry in Children

Editors

JOHN H. HERMAN
MAX HIRSHKOWITZ

SLEEP MEDICINE CLINICS

www.sleep.theclinics.com

Consulting Editor
TEOFILO LEE-CHIONG Jr

June 2015 • Volume 10 • Number 2

ELSEVIER

1600 John F. Kennedy Boulevard ● Suite 1800 ● Philadelphia, Pennsylvania, 19103-2899

http://www.theclinics.com

SLEEP MEDICINE CLINICS Volume 10, Number 2
June 2015, ISSN 1556-407X, ISBN-13: 978-0-323-38906-8

Editor: Patrick Manley
Developmental Editor: Donald Mumford

Sleep Medicine Clinics (ISSN 1556-407X) is published quarterly by Elsevier Inc., 360 Park Avenue South, New York, NY 10010-1710. Months of issue are March, June, September and December. Business and Editorial Offices: 1600 John F. Kennedy Blvd., Ste. 1800, Philadelphia, PA 19103-2899. Customer Service Office: 3251 Riverport Lane, Maryland Heights, MO 63043. Periodicals postage paid at New York, NY and additional mailing offices. Subscription prices are $195.00 per year (US individuals), $95.00 (US residents), $406.00 (US institutions), $230.00 (Canadian individuals), $235.00 (international individuals), $135.00 (Canadian and international residents) and $452.00 (Canadian and international institutions). Foreign air speed delivery is included in all *Clinics* subscription prices. All prices are subject to change without notice. **POSTMASTER:** Send change of address to *Sleep Medicine Clinics*, Elsevier Health Sciences Division, Subscription Customer Service, 3251 Riverport Lane, Maryland Heights, MO 63043. Customer Service: **Tel: 1-800-654-2452 (U.S. and Canada); 314-447-8871 (outside U.S. and Canada). Fax: 314-447-8029. E-mail: journalscustomerservice-usa@elsevier.com (for print support); journalsonline support-usa@elsevier.com (for online support).**

Reprints. For copies of 100 or more of articles in this publication, please contact the Commercial Reprints Department, Elsevier Inc., 360 Park Avenue South, New York, NY 10010-1710. Tel.: 212-633-3874; Fax: 212-633-3820; E-mail: reprints@elsevier.com.

Sleep Medicine Clinics is covered in *MEDLINE/PubMed (Index Medicus).*

PROGRAM OBJECTIVE

The goal of *Sleep Clinics of North America* is to keep practicing physicians up to date with current clinical practice by providing timely articles reviewing the state of the art in patient care.

TARGET AUDIENCE

All practicing physicians and other healthcare professionals.

LEARNING OBJECTIVES

Upon completion of this activity, participants will be able to:
1. Review the relationship between sleep and mental health in children.
2. Discuss the comorbidity of sleep disorders and behavioural-psychiatric syndromes in paediatrics.
3. Recognize the effects of sleep disorders on children's emotions and cognitive functions.

ACCREDITATION

The Elsevier Office of Continuing Medical Education (EOCME) is accredited by the Accreditation Council for Continuing Medical Education (ACCME) to provide continuing medical education for physicians.

The EOCME designates this enduring material for a maximum of 15 *AMA PRA Category 1 Credit*(s)™. Physicians should claim only the credit commensurate with the extent of their participation in the activity.

All other health care professionals requesting continuing education credit for this enduring material will be issued a certificate of participation.

DISCLOSURE OF CONFLICTS OF INTEREST

The EOCME assesses conflict of interest with its instructors, faculty, planners, and other individuals who are in a position to control the content of CME activities. All relevant conflicts of interest that are identified are thoroughly vetted by EOCME for fair balance, scientific objectivity, and patient care recommendations. EOCME is committed to providing its learners with CME activities that promote improvements or quality in healthcare and not a specific proprietary business or a commercial interest.

The planning committee, staff, authors and editors listed below have identified no financial relationships or relationships to products or devices they or their spouse/life partner have with commercial interest related to the content of this CME activity:

Candice A. Alfano, PhD; Isabelle Arnulf, MD, PhD; Penny Corkum, PhD; Fiona Davidson, MA; Anjali Fortna; Michael Gradisar, PhD; Alice M. Gregory, BA, PhD; Kristen Helm; John H. Herman, PhD; Max Hirshkowitz, PhD; Suresh Kotagal, MD; Beth A. Malow, MD, MS; Patrick Manley; Mahalakshmi Narayanan; Louise M. O'Brien, PhD, MS; Katharine C. Reynolds, MA; Ralph E. Schmidt, PhD; A.J. Schwichtenberg, PhD; Martial Van der Linden, PhD; Jennifer Vriend, PhD; Thomas A. Willis, BSc, PhD.

The planning committee, staff, authors and editors listed below have identified financial relationships or relationships to products or devices they or their spouse/life partner have with commercial interest related to the content of this CME activity:

Benjamin Rusak, PhD, FRSC is a consultant/advisor for the Institut de Recherches Internationales Servier, of DDMoRe.
Teofilo Lee-Chiong Jr, MD has stock ownership, a research grant and an employment affiliation with Koninklijke Philips N.V.; is a consultant/advisor for CareCore National and Elsevier; and has royalties/patents with Elsevier, Lippincott, Wiley, Oxford University and CreateSpace.

UNAPPROVED/OFF-LABEL USE DISCLOSURE

The EOCME requires CME faculty to disclose to the participants:
1. When products or procedures being discussed are off-label, unlabelled, experimental, and/or investigational (not US Food and Drug Administration [FDA] approved); and
2. Any limitations on the information presented, such as data that are preliminary or that represent ongoing research, interim analyses, and/or unsupported opinions. Faculty may discuss information about pharmaceutical agents that is outside of FDA-approved labelling. This information is intended solely for CME and is not intended to promote off-label use of these medications. If you have any questions, contact the medical affairs department of the manufacturer for the most recent prescribing information.

TO ENROLL

To enroll in the Sleep Medicines Clinic Continuing Medical Education program, call customer service at 1-800-654-2452 or sign up online at http://www.theclinics.com/home/cme. The CME program is available to subscribers for an additional annual fee of USD $140.

METHOD OF PARTICIPATION

In order to claim credit, participants must complete the following:
1. Complete enrolment as indicated above.
2. Read the activity.

3. Complete the CME Test and Evaluation. Participants must achieve a score of 70% on the test. All CME Tests and Evaluations must be completed online.

CME INQUIRIES/SPECIAL NEEDS
For all CME inquiries or special needs, please contact elsevierCME@elsevier.com.

SLEEP MEDICINE CLINICS

FORTHCOMING ISSUES

September 2015
Restless Legs Syndrome and Movement Disorders
Denise Sharon, *Editor*

December 2015
Science of Circadian Rhythms
Phyllis Zee, *Editor*

March 2016
Sleep in Medical and Neurologic Disorders
Flavia Consens, *Editor*

RECENT ISSUES

March 2015
Sleep and Psychiatry in Adults
John Herman and Max Hirshkowitz, *Editors*

December 2014
Evaluation of Sleep Complaints
Clete A. Kushida, *Editor*

September 2014
Sleep Hypoventilation: A State-of-the-Art Overview
Babak Mokhlesi, *Editor*

ISSUES OF RELATED INTEREST

Clinics in Chest Medicine, Vol. 35, No.3 (September 2014)
Sleep-Disordered Breathing: Beyond Obstructive Sleep Apnea
Carolyn M. D'Ambrosio, *Editor*

THE CLINICS ARE AVAILABLE ONLINE!
Access your subscription at:
www.theclinics.com

Contributors

CONSULTING EDITOR

TEOFILO LEE-CHIONG Jr, MD
Professor of Medicine, National Jewish Health;
Professor of Medicine, School of Medicine,
University of Colorado Denver, Denver,
Colorado; Chief Medical Liaison, Philips
Respironics, Pennsylvania

EDITORS

JOHN H. HERMAN, PhD
Adjunct Professor of Psychiatry and Pediatrics,
University of Texas Southwestern Medical
Center at Dallas, Dallas, Texas

MAX HIRSHKOWITZ, PhD
Professor Emeritus, Baylor College of
Medicine, Houston, Texas; Consulting
Professor, Stanford University School of
Medicine, Palo Alto, California

AUTHORS

CANDICE A. ALFANO, PhD
Associate Professor of Psychology, Sleep and
Anxiety Center of Houston, Department of
Psychology, University of Houston, Houston,
Texas

ISABELLE ARNULF, MD, PhD
Professor, Sleep Disorder Unit, National
Reference Center for Narcolepsy, Idiopathic
Hypersomnia and Kleine Levin Syndrome,
Inserm, Pitié-Salpêtrière Hospital (APHP), Paris
6 University, Paris, France

PENNY CORKUM, PhD
Registered Psychologist, Professor,
Department of Psychology and Neuroscience,
Dalhousie University, Halifax, Nova Scotia,
Canada

FIONA DAVIDSON, MA
Clinical Psychology PhD Student, Department
of Psychology and Neuroscience, Dalhousie
University, Halifax, Nova Scotia, Canada

MICHAEL GRADISAR, PhD
Associate Professor in Clinical Child
Psychology, School of Psychology, Flinders
University, Adelaide, South Australia, Australia

ALICE M. GREGORY, BA, PhD
Reader in Psychology, Department of
Psychology, Goldsmiths, University of London,
London, United Kingdom

JOHN H. HERMAN, PhD
Adjunct Professor of Psychiatry and Pediatrics,
University of Texas Southwestern Medical
Center at Dallas, Dallas, Texas

SURESH KOTAGAL, MD
Division of Child Neurology, Mayo Clinic,
Rochester, Minnesota

BETH A. MALOW, MD, MS
Burry Chair in Cognitive Childhood
Development; Director, Sleep Disorders
Division; Professor, Department of Neurology,
Vanderbilt University Medical Center,
Nashville, Tennessee

LOUISE M. O'BRIEN, PhD, MS
Associate Professor, Department of
Neurology, Sleep Disorders Center;
Associate Research Scientist,
Department of Oral and Maxillofacial
Surgery, University of Michigan,
Ann Arbor, Michigan

KATHARINE C. REYNOLDS, MA
Clinical Psychology Graduate Student, Sleep and Anxiety Center of Houston, Department of Psychology, University of Houston, Houston, Texas

BENJAMIN RUSAK, PhD, FRSC
Professor and Director of Research, Department of Psychiatry; Professor of Psychology and Neuroscience and Pharmacology, Departments of Psychology and Neuroscience, Psychiatry, and Pharmacology, Dalhousie University, Halifax, Nova Scotia, Canada

RALPH E. SCHMIDT, PhD
Swiss Center for Affective Sciences, Department of Psychology, University of Geneva; Cognitive Psychopathology and Neuropsychology Unit, Department of Psychology, University of Geneva, Geneva, Switzerland

A.J. SCHWICHTENBERG, PhD
Assistant Professor, Department of Human Development and Family Studies; Department of Psychological Sciences; Department of Speech, Language, and Hearing Sciences, Purdue University, West Lafayette, Indiana

MARTIAL VAN DER LINDEN, PhD
Swiss Center for Affective Sciences, Department of Psychology, University of Geneva; Cognitive Psychopathology and Neuropsychology Unit, Department of Psychology, University of Geneva, Geneva, Switzerland

JENNIFER VRIEND, PhD
Registered Psychologist, Queensview Professional Services, Ottawa, Ontario, Canada

THOMAS A. WILLIS, BSc, PhD
Research Fellow, Leeds Institute of Health Sciences, University of Leeds, Leeds, United Kingdom

Contents

Preface: Sleep Medicine and Psychiatric Disorders in Children   xiii

John H. Herman and Max Hirshkowitz

Emotional and Cognitive Impact of Sleep Restriction in Children   107

Jennifer Vriend, Fiona Davidson, Benjamin Rusak, and Penny Corkum

Several observational, cross-sectional, and longitudinal studies as well as a few well-controlled experimental studies have examined the impact of sleep loss on children's daytime functioning. The emerging results indicate that sleep plays a critical role in various aspects of daytime functioning in children, including cognitive and emotional functioning. Furthermore, studies indicate that daytime functioning may be impaired by even small amounts of sleep restriction in children.

The Relations Between Sleep, Personality, Behavioral Problems, and School Performance in Adolescents   117

Ralph E. Schmidt and Martial Van der Linden

According to recent meta-analyses, adolescents across different countries and cultures do not get the recommended amount of sleep. Extracurricular activities, part-time jobs, and use of electronic devices in the evening delay bedtime in adolescents. Early school start times also shorten the time for sleep. Insufficient sleep in adolescents has been associated with weakened emotional-behavioral regulation and poor academic achievement. Multicomponent intervention programs have been developed on the basis of cognitive-behavioral therapy for insomnia to improve sleep in youth.

Anxiety Disorders and Sleep in Children and Adolescents   125

Thomas A. Willis and Alice M. Gregory

Sleep problems are common in children and adolescents. A growing body of research has explored the relationship between sleep problems and anxiety in youth. When reviewing the literature, methodologic inconsistencies need to be considered, such as variation in conceptualization of sleep problems, measurement of sleep, and the classification of anxiety. Despite this, there seems to be good evidence of concurrent and longitudinal associations between sleep difficulties and anxiety in community and clinical samples of young people. Potential mechanisms are proposed. There is a need for further exploration of these relationships, with the hope of aiding preventive capability and developing useful treatments.

Sleep in Children and Adolescents with Obsessive-Compulsive Disorder   133

Katharine C. Reynolds, Michael Gradisar, and Candice A. Alfano

Sleep problems are not a core feature of obsessive-compulsive disorder (OCD), but emerging empirical data indicate some form of sleep disruption to be highly common. Available research in both adult and child patients is limited in several important ways, including the use of subjective reports (particularly in children), high rates of comorbid depression, and concurrent use of psychotropic medication. The presence of sleep disruption in OCD patients may compound severity and impairment of the disorder. More research is needed to fully understand the nature and consequences of sleep-wake disruption in children with OCD.

Attention Deficit/Hyperactivity Disorder and Sleep in Children   143

John H. Herman

Basic assumptions about ADHD in children and sleep are not supported by research. It is unclear that children with hyperactivity or inattention have disrupted sleep. Parents of children with ADHD consistently report more bedtime resistance, but there is no objective evidence that sleep is subsequently disrupted. Treatment of ADHD with stimulants may disrupt sleep. Studies of comorbid sleep or psychiatric disorders consistently show that they disrupt sleep. Melatonin is an effective treatment of sleep problems in children with ADHD. Before any child is placed on stimulants, the pediatrician or other health care professional should insure that the child is obtaining adequate sleep.

Kleine-Levin Syndrome   151

Isabelle Arnulf

Kleine-Levin syndrome is a rare recurrent encephalopathy primarily affecting teenagers, characterized by relapsing-remitting episodes of hypersomnia along with cognitive, psychiatric and behavioral disturbances. During episodes, patients suddenly present hypersomnia (with sleep lasting 15-21 h/d), cognitive impairment (major apathy, confusion, slowness, amnesia), and a specific feeling of derealization (dreamy state, altered perception). Less frequently, they may also experience hyperphagia (66%), hypersexuality (53%, principally men), depressed mood (53%, principally women), anxiety, hallucinations, and acute brief psychosis (33%). Brain functional imaging is often abnormal. Stimulants are poorly beneficial during episodes, whereas lithium and valproate help reducing the episodes frequency and duration.

Rapid Eye Movement Sleep Behavior Disorder During Childhood   163

Suresh Kotagal

Rapid eye movement (REM) sleep behavior disorder (RBD) is a type of parasomnia that arises out of REM sleep and is characterized by aggressive or violent motor dream enactment in conjunction with preservation of tonic electromyographic activity (ie, REM sleep without atonia). RBD occurs at all ages and in both sexes, although it remains relatively infrequent during childhood. The literature pertaining to RBD in childhood is scant, and composed only of single case reports or small case series. RBD etiologies include Parkinson disease, multisystem atrophy, and dementia with Lewy body disease. This article presents an updated review of childhood RBD.

Sleep-Related Breathing Disorder, Cognitive Functioning, and Behavioral-Psychiatric Syndromes in Children   169

Louise M. O'Brien

Childhood sleep disordered breathing (SDB) is strongly associated with a range of cognitive and behavioral disturbances, including some psychiatric diagnoses. Despite this, the majority of children with symptoms of SDB go unrecognized, even though simple screening could identify children in need of further evaluation. Definitive evidence showing that SDB causes cognitive and behavioral impairment has yet to emerge, although a randomized controlled trial evaluating neuropsychological and health outcomes of treatment for SDB in children is currently underway.

Melatonin Treatment in Children with Developmental Disabilities   181

A.J. Schwichtenberg and Beth A. Malow

Melatonin is commonly recommended to treat sleep problems in children with developmental disabilities. However, few studies document the efficacy and safety of melatonin in these populations. This article reviews recent studies of melatonin efficacy in developmental disabilities. Overall, short treatment trials were associated with a significant decrease in sleep onset latency time for each of the disorders reviewed, with 1 notable exception—tuberous sclerosis. Reported side effects were uncommon and mild. Across disorders, additional research is needed to draw disability-specific conclusions. However, studies to date provide positive support for future trials that include larger groups of children with specific disabilities/syndromes.

Preface

Sleep Medicine and Psychiatric Disorders in Children

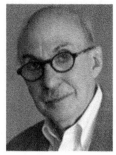 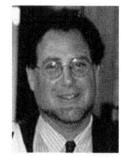

John H. Herman, PhD   Max Hirshkowitz, PhD

Editors

From birth to adolescence, an individual traverses a remarkable path during which developmental changes alter every aspect of mind and body. This change far exceeds what will occur in the remainder of life. The developing brain undergoes such remarkable and rapid maturation that the amorphous brain waves present at birth are scored as "infant sleep." After the first six months, adult brain waves have emerged and adult sleep stages can be scored. Thereafter, sleep stage scoring according to guidelines of the American Academy of Sleep Medicine remains consistent throughout the life span.

Sleep requirements undergo equally momentous changes, from the sleep depth and duration observed in a newborn to an adult-like pattern emerging in late adolescence. Sleep-need rapidly changes. Newborns sleep most of the day and night at a depth immune to most attempts to disturb them. By late adolescence, sleep might be disrupted much like an adult.

Many psychiatric disorders and sleep disorders develop early in life, frequently in parallel fashion. This issue focuses on the relationship between these disorders and how each might influence the other. For example, children who develop psychiatric disorders exhibit more disrupted sleep than age-matched normal controls.[1] Likewise, disrupted sleep in young children (without sleep restriction) correlates with subsequent sleepiness and cognitive dysfunction.[2]

This issue opens with an article by Vriend and Davidson demonstrating frailty in children confronted with mild sleep restriction (1 hour) with respect to both emotion and cognition. Schmidt and coworkers then review evidence indicating that sleep quality in adolescents correlates with personality characteristics, behavioral problems, and quality of school performance. These two articles demonstrate the need for adequate sleep during development to support cognitive, behavioral, and emotional functioning.

Subsequent articles focus on specific psychiatric or sleep disorders in children. We review the evidence associating the spectrum of anxiety disorders with disrupted sleep in children and adolescents (Willis). The relationship between obsessive compulsive disorder and childhood insomnia is explored in the ensuing article (Reynolds et al). The next article addresses the complex relationship between attention deficit hyperactivity disorder and sleep. It also addresses the question

Sleep Med Clin 10 (2015) xiii–xiv
http://dx.doi.org/10.1016/j.jsmc.2015.04.001
1556-407X/15/$ – see front matter © 2015 Published by Elsevier Inc.

of cause and effect. These three articles offer significant evidence relating disrupted sleep in childhood to specific behavioral, emotional, and psychiatric disorders.

Kleine-Levin syndrome is a rare, episodic disorder of hypersomnolence. We included a meta-analysis by Arnulf of existing literature (both from a descriptive and treatment perspective) to highlight this sleep disorder's dramatic behavioral effects. Dr Kortugal then reviews evidence connecting REM sleep behavioral disorder in children to neurodevelopmental disabilities. No discussion of sleep disorders is complete without considering obstructive sleep apnea. We therefore included the description by O'Brien and colleagues of the relationship between obstructive sleep apnea syndrome and cognitive, behavioral, and psychiatric disabilities in children. We conclude with Schwich-tenberg and Malow's finding that treating developmental disabilities with melatonin has limited efficacy, but in many cases is still of value.

We hope this issue will prove useful to practitioners and researchers interested in pediatric sleep and psychiatric disorders. Sleep disorders are clinically underserved and understanding their relationship with psychiatric problems would benefit from better recognition. Similarly, sleep alterations associated with psychiatric disorders can produce a synergistic downward spiral in health and well-being.

John H. Herman, PhD
University of Texas
Southwestern Medical Center at Dallas
Dallas, TX, USA

Max Hirshkowitz, PhD
Baylor College of Medicine
Houston, TX, USA

Stanford University School of Medicine
Palo Alto, CA, USA

E-mail addresses:
john.herman.phd@gmail.com (J.H. Herman)
max.hirshkowitz@gmail.com (M. Hirshkowitz)

REFERENCES

1. Lunsford-Avery JR, Orr JM, Gupta T, et al. Sleep dysfunction and thalamic abnormalities in adolescents at ultra high-risk for psychosis. Schizophr Res 2013;151(1–3):148–53.
2. Ramesh V, Nair D, Zhang SX, et al. Disrupted sleep without sleep curtailment induces sleepiness and cognitive dysfunction via the tumor necrosis factor-α pathway. J Neuroinflammation 2012;9:91.

Emotional and Cognitive Impact of Sleep Restriction in Children

Jennifer Vriend, PhD[a], Fiona Davidson, MA[b],
Benjamin Rusak, PhD, FRSC[c,d,e], Penny Corkum, PhD[b,*]

KEYWORDS

- Sleep restriction • Daytime functioning • Cognitive functioning • Emotional functioning

KEY POINTS

- Evidence is mounting to suggest that sleep restriction in the pediatric population has marked negative effects.
- Inadequate quantity and quality of sleep are associated with various impairments in daytime functioning.
- Studies reveal that even moderate amounts of sleep restriction over just a few days impair aspects of emotional and cognitive functioning.
- A few hypotheses have been advanced to explain how sleep restriction affects daytime functioning in adults, but these have not been assessed in the pediatric population.
- The high prevalence of poor sleep and the multitude of negative consequences emphasize the need for increased public awareness about the importance of sleep and the value of early identification and treatment of sleep problems in children.

INTRODUCTION

Approximately 30 years ago, Carskadon and colleagues[1] conducted seminal studies examining the effects of sleep loss in children. In addition to finding impairments in some areas of daytime functioning after sleep restriction, they also found that children might not recover from sleep restriction as rapidly as adults. Since that time, several observational, cross-sectional, and longitudinal studies, as well as a few well-controlled experimental studies, have been published, and the emerging results indicate that sleep plays a critical role in the regulation of cognitive and emotional functioning in children.

The goals of this article are to review the current pediatric literature examining sleep restriction effects on daytime functioning, highlight the general findings, and pose questions to direct future research. The impact of poor sleep on daytime sleepiness, emotional functioning, and cognitive functioning is reviewed first. Then 3 hypotheses, derived from the adult literature, are introduced about how sleep restriction affects daytime functioning, and the extent to which they can be applied to children is reviewed, based on the pediatric literature. The results of experimental sleep restriction studies conducted in the pediatric population are highlighted (**Table 1** has an overview of these studies). This article concludes by

[a] Queensview Professional Services, 600-2725 Queensview Avenue, Ottawa, Ontario K2B 0A1, Canada;
[b] Department of Psychology & Neuroscience, Dalhousie University, 1355 Oxford Street, PO BOX 15000, Halifax, Nova Scotia B3H 4R2, Canada; [c] Department of Psychiatry, Dalhousie University, 5909 Veterans Memorial Lane, Halifax, Nova Scotia B3H 2E2, Canada; [d] Department of Psychology & Neuroscience, Dalhousie University, 5909 Veterans Memorial Lane, Halifax, Nova Scotia B3H 2E2, Canada; [e] Department of Pharmacology, Dalhousie University, 5909 Veterans Memorial Lane, Halifax, Nova Scotia B3H 2E2, Canada
* Corresponding author.
E-mail address: penny.corkum@dal.ca

Sleep Med Clin 10 (2015) 107–115
http://dx.doi.org/10.1016/j.jsmc.2015.02.009
1556-407X/15/$ – see front matter © 2015 Elsevier Inc. All rights reserved.

Table 1
Summary of the studies examining the effects of sleep restriction on emotional and cognitive functioning in school-aged children

Study	Participants/Age	Design	Sleep Restriction Protocol	Findings
Carskadon et al, 1981a	12 Participants (11–15 y; 67% boys)	Within-participants	No sleep for 1 night compared with 10 h time in bed for 1 night	Objective (MSLT) and subjective sleepiness increased. Performance on addition and memory tasks were impaired in sleep restriction condition.
Carskadon et al, 1981b	9 Participants (11–13 y; 33% boys)	Within-participants	4 h Time in bed for 1 night compared with 10 h time in bed for 1 night	Objective sleepiness (MSLT) increased. No significant changes on cognitive tasks.
Randazzo et al, 1998	16 Participants (10–14 y; 44% boys)	Between-participants (8 per group)	5 h In bed for 1 night compared with 11 h in bed for 1 night	Sleep restriction impaired performance on 3 measures of creativity and a measure of reasoning. Nine other measures of cognitive performance were not affected.
Fallone et al, 2001	82 Participants (8–15 y; 49% boys)	Between-participants (37 sleep-extended; 45 sleep-restricted)	4 h Time in bed compared with 10 h time in bed	Sleep restriction increased objective (MSLT) and subjective sleepiness and inattentive behaviors (RA-rated) but not hyper/impulsive behaviors. No differences were found on objective tests of attention.
Sadeh et al, 2003	77 Participants (9–12 y; unknown gender distribution)	Mixed within- and between-participants (21 sleep-extended; 28 sleep-restricted; 23 no sleep change)	2 Nights of normal sleep and 3 nights of ± 1 h difference in normal sleep duration	Extended sleep led to improved memory function and CPT performance, and maintained performance on a simple reaction time test.
Fallone et al, 2005	74 Participants (6–12 y; 53% boys)	Within-participants	6.5–8 h Per night for 1 wk compared with 10+ h per night for 1 wk and compared with baseline week of self-selected sleep	Sleep restriction increased teacher-reported sleepiness, academic problems, and inattention.

Study	Participants	Design	Sleep condition	Findings
Peters et al, 2009	14 (10 y; 100% girls)	Within-participants	Sleep restriction (5 h time in bed) compared with control (10 h time in bed)	Sleep restriction was associated with longer average response times and increased number of lapses.
Talbot et al, 2010	20 Young adolescents (10–13 y), 24 midadolescents (13–16 y), and 20 adults (30–60 y)	Within-participants	Maximum of 6.5 h total sleep time on 1st night followed by a maximum of 2 h total sleep time on 2nd night. The rested condition was approximately 7–8 h total sleep time for 2 nights.	Fewer positive affects was observed in the sleep-deprived, compared with rested. Participants also reported a greater increase in anxiety during a catastrophizing task. Additionally, early adolescents rated their main worry as more threatening when sleep deprived compared with rested.
Gruber et al, 2011	43 Participants (7–11 y; 64% boys); 32 TD and 11 children with ADHD	Within-participants	1 h Less than typical time in bed for 6 nights compared with typical time in bed	Sleep restriction led to poorer CPT scores on 2/3 of CPT measures in TD children and children with ADHD.
Vriend et al, 2013	32 Participants (8–12 y; 44% boys)	Within-participants	1 h Less than typical time in bed compared with 1 h more than typical time in bed	Sleep restriction, compared with extension and led to poorer short-term and working memory, divided attention, parent-reported attention, emotion regulation, and positive affective response.

Abbreviations: ADHD, attention-deficit/hyperactivity disorder; CPT, continuous performance test; MSLT, multiple sleep latency test; RA, research assistant; TD, typically developing.

emphasizing the need to increase public awareness about the importance of sleep and the value of early identification and treatment of sleep problems in children.

POOR SLEEP AND SLEEPINESS

Not surprisingly, sleepiness is the clearest and most consistent result of sleep restriction.[1,2] Sleepiness in children and youth is common, with many high school students and teachers suggesting in surveys that falling asleep in school is a common behavior.[3] One study found that an 85-minute delay in high school start times resulted in youth getting approximately 5 hours more sleep per week, showing reduced sleeping in class.[4] Much of the focus on sleepiness in children has targeted adolescent populations. There is also evidence to suggest, however, that reductions in sleep time result in increased sleepiness in younger school-aged populations.[1,5] For example, Carskadon and colleagues[1] found that after 1 night of sleep restriction, sleep-onset latencies dropped from an average of 15 minutes to below 5 minutes, indicating severe sleepiness. Other studies have shown that even moderate reductions in sleep duration result in increased sleepiness as assessed using objective sleep measures.[6]

POOR SLEEP AND EMOTIONAL FUNCTIONING

Understanding the impact of sleep on emotional functioning in children is important because childhood is a critical stage during which children develop their ability to regulate emotions.[7] Several naturalistic studies have examined sleep in children with a variety of clinical conditions and found poor sleep to be associated with anxiety,[8,9] emotional problems,[10] and depressive symptoms.[11] Johnson and colleagues[12] investigated the order of appearance of insomnia, anxiety, and depression in adolescents. Retrospective reports showed that anxiety disorders preceded insomnia in 73% of comorbid cases whereas insomnia preceded depression in 69% of comorbid cases.

Only a few studies have used objective measures to examine sleep and emotional functioning in children with psychological disorders. Bertocci and colleagues[13] compared polysomnographic (PSG) recordings from children with depression with those from healthy control children. Although depressed youth reported significantly worse sleep in terms of quality and awakenings, PSG measures indicated no evidence of disturbed sleep in the depressed sample compared with controls. Also using PSG, Forbes and colleagues[14] found that individuals with anxiety have poorer sleep than either controls or those with depression. Another study found that children with anxiety slept for shorter periods than children in an age- and gender-matched control group.[15] Sadeh and colleagues[16] found that children's self-ratings of depression, hopelessness, and low self-esteem were significantly correlated with poorer sleep quality as measured by actigraphy. Several longitudinal studies have also demonstrated that sleep problems in early childhood predict later emotional problems and the emergence of psychological disorders.[17,18] These studies indicate that sleep problems in early life reflect processes leading to the emergence of disorders of emotional regulation or actually contribute to their emergence.

Even fewer studies have used objective measures to examine sleep and emotional functioning in nonclinical populations, but evidence is accumulating that even for otherwise healthy children, inadequate sleep may have negative consequences for emotional regulation. Aronen and colleagues[19] studied 49 healthy children and found significant associations between shorter total sleep time, as measured by actigraphy, and higher teacher ratings of externalizing behavior, inattention, and social problems. Vriend and colleagues[20] found that in a group of typically developing 8- to 12-year-old children, shorter sleep duration was significantly associated with higher levels of negative affective response.

Although many researchers have suggested an association between problematic sleep and negative emotional functioning, only 2 studies[21,22] have demonstrated a causal relation between short sleep and changes in emotional regulation by examining the effects of experimentally manipulating sleep duration in pediatric populations. Talbot and colleagues[21] and Vriend and colleagues[22] both found that reducing sleep duration resulted in reduced positive affect without a change in levels of negative affect. Talbot and colleagues[21] also reported that young adolescents expressed more anxiety when engaged in a task related to catastrophizing and endorsed a higher likelihood of a catastrophic event when sleep restricted relative to a well-rested control condition.

Whereas Talbot and colleagues[21] studied young adolescents during the mornings after a 2-hour sleep opportunity, Vriend and colleagues[22] compared the effects of sleep extension and restriction over 4 nights in each condition that resulted in only approximately 1-hour differences in nightly sleep duration. These small reductions in sleep duration over only 4 nights reduced positive affect and the ability to regulate emotion. More severe and sustained sleep loss could contribute to the emergence of, or perpetuate, disorders of emotional regulation, including depression and anxiety.

POOR SLEEP AND COGNITIVE FUNCTIONING

Most of the research on cognitive functioning and sleep in children has been based on surveys indicating that irregular sleep-wake patterns are associated with poor academic achievement[23] or correlational studies reporting that early school start times are associated with poor academic performance.[3] For example, 1 study[4] followed 12,000 youths for 2 years before and 3 years after an 85-minute delay in school start times. They found that later school start times resulted in decreased tardiness, increased graduation rates, improved academic performance, and higher morale. One study found that children with academic and/or attention problems in school are more likely to have sleep problems compared with children who are not experiencing such problems.[24] Another study found that morning cognitive performance was poor in children whose spontaneous self-reported sleep the previous night was either shorter or longer than their typical sleep.[25]

A few studies have used objective measures of sleep (ie, actigraphy and PSG) to examine the relationships between sleep quantity and efficiency and cognitive variables in children. Using actigraphy, these studies have found correlations between impaired cognitive functioning and poor sleep quality[20,26,27] as well as short sleep duration.[28]

Experimental research is critical to understanding the daytime consequences of inadequate sleep, because causality can only be inferred from these types of studies. Although no studies have examined the effect of experimentally fragmenting sleep (ie, waking children during the night) on cognitive functioning in children, several studies have looked at the effects of experimentally restricting sleep duration on cognitive functioning in school-aged children. Among these studies, 8 reported negative effects of sleep reduction on some aspects of cognitive functioning but not on other aspects,[1,2,5,6,29–32] whereas 1 did not report any significant impairment.[33] The studies reporting impaired functioning after sleep loss identified deficits in several domains, such as addition tasks and word memory tasks[1]; verbal creativity, learning new abstract concepts, and abstract thinking[6]; teacher-reported academic problems and severity of attention problems[29]; research assistant–reported

inattention[2]; simple reaction time[5]; and vigilance and sustained attention.[30,31]

Beebe and colleagues[34,35] conducted studies examining the effects of sleep restriction on slightly older adolescents (approximately 14–17 years). They found that when participants were sleep restricted, parents reported that the adolescents had significantly greater problems with sleepiness, attention, oppositionality/irritability, behavior regulation, metacognition, and simulated classroom performance. Participant self-reports indicated similar but less robust results. Beebe and colleagues[36] found that in adolescents who were sleep restricted, regions of the brain that are normally active during an attention-demanding, working memory task showed greater activation, whereas brain areas that are normally suppressed during attention-demanding tasks showed even greater suppression. The investigators hypothesized that this response was a compensatory strategy to help individuals focus their attention after chronic sleep restriction.

MECHANISMS MEDIATING SLEEP LOSS EFFECTS

Together the studies (discussed previously) provide evidence that certain areas of cognitive functioning are impaired by poor or inadequate sleep. These results are consistent with the adult literature on sleep loss and cognitive functioning (see Walker[37] for review). The pediatric literature includes few attempts to analyze the mechanisms by which sleep loss modulates emotional and cognitive functioning. To help guide thinking about these issues in the pediatric population, the 3 main hypotheses that have been discussed in the adult literature related to sleep loss and cognitive function are reviewed.

These hypotheses are the vigilance hypothesis, the neuropsychological hypothesis, and the controlled attention hypothesis (for review, see Lim and Dinges[38]). Because both adult and pediatric research studies of sleep effects on daytime function have focused principally on cognitive consequences, these hypotheses have been developed primarily to address mechanisms related to the effects of sleep loss on cognition.

The Vigilance Hypothesis

Several investigators have suggested that decrements in performance are simply due to a general decrease in arousal and vigilance. Supporters of this hypothesis suggest that sleep loss affects nearly all cognitive capacities in a global manner through lowered vigilance and alertness.[39] Balkin and colleagues[40(p654)] summarize this view by stating, "sleep loss impacts a wide array of cognitive abilities. In fact, the array is so extensive that it is reasonable to posit that sleep loss exerts a nonspecific effect on cognitive performance." Few researchers have addressed whether the nonspecific vigilance hypothesis might also apply to emotional functioning. It could be hypothesized that a general reduction in arousal after sleep loss might lead to a decrease in emotional responses, especially to stimuli eliciting positive responses.[41] This interpretation is consistent with the results of Talbot and colleagues[21] and Vriend and colleagues,[22] in that sleep restriction in children reduced positive affective responses but did not increase negative affective responses. Another study reported that sleep loss in medical residents dampened responses to positive opportunities while amplifying negative feelings and fatigue in response to negative daytime events; these responses were related to reduced availability of cognitive energy for responding to either class of events.[42] This interpretation may be seen as related to a general lowering of arousal after sleep loss but with an increase in negativity and fatigue associated with daytime disruptions. Whether sleep loss intensifies negative feelings may depend on the nature of the circumstances giving rise to these feelings: sleep-restricted children viewing negative visual images may respond differently from medical residents dealing with negative events during their work day.

The Neuropsychological Hypothesis

Harrison and Horne[43] proposed a neuropsychological model based on recent neuroimaging and clinical data. They suggested that sleep deprivation might affect performance negatively due to a decrease in activity in the prefrontal cortex (PFC). According to this hypothesis, tasks that place heavy demands on the PFC are most vulnerable to sleep restriction.

Not all of the functions of the PFC are known, but key functions include the maintenance of wakefulness and nonspecific arousal, decision making, innovative thinking, response inhibition, revising plans, attending selectively, and effective communication.[43] Some areas of the PFC are critically involved in regulating behavior and mood as well as in performing cognitive tasks. Thus, impairments in cognitive and emotional functions after sleep loss may share a common pathophysiologic mechanism related to PFC activity.[44]

The involvement of the PFC in mood regulation includes inhibiting limbic structures, such as the amygdala and the hippocampus, that play important roles in both generating and recognizing affective states.[45–47] Neuroimaging studies in adults indicate that sleep restriction leads to greater amygdala responses to negative emotional stimuli[48] and weaker connectivity between the medial PFC and the amygdala,[49] resulting in problems moderating emotional responses.

Based on this hypothesis, impairments after sleep loss are expected on more complex cognitive tasks, such as working memory, executive attention, and divided attention, that depend heavily on PFC function. Several studies have suggested that more complex cognitive tasks are most vulnerable to sleep restriction,[6] whereas others have found that some complex tasks are not affected. As suggested in the adult literature, it is likely that specific task characteristics and/or participant characteristics influence the sensitivity of different tasks to sleep-related impairments.

The Controlled Attention Hypothesis

Somewhat in contrast to predictions from the neuropsychological hypothesis, some studies have found that highly demanding tasks are unaffected by sleep restriction.[50,51] These results have been interpreted using a controlled attention model.[52] These investigators suggest that tasks that are monotonous, boring, and/or intrinsically less engaging are more affected by sleep restriction because greater (more effortful) top-down control is needed to sustain optimal performance. Pilcher and colleagues[52] suggested that tasks should be classified based on whether they encourage attentive behaviors, with tasks that are low on this dimension the most likely to be affected by sleep restriction, whereas tasks that encourage a high degree of attention and engagement the least affected by sleep restriction.

Both the neuropsychological and controlled attention hypotheses predict that tasks requiring more top-down control, such as regulation of emotional responses, are strongly affected by sleep loss. Yoo and colleagues,[49] for example, suggested that sleep deprivation increased negative emotions due to a failure of top-down, prefrontal control. Similarly, boring and less engaging tasks that require top-down input to maintain performance should also be strongly affected by sleep loss. Some studies reported, however, that monotonous and less engaging tasks were not affected by sleep restriction.[2,22] Perhaps a moderate amount of task engagement is necessary for a task to be sensitive to the effects of sleep restriction.

Summary of Hypotheses

The 3 hypotheses (discussed previously) are not mutually incompatible. For example, Lim and

Dinges[38] suggested that the vigilance and controlled attention hypotheses could be viewed as different explanations of the same set of phenomena. The published adult literature provides support for and against all of these hypotheses, so there is no consensus around any model to account for the role of sleep in daytime functioning. Given the limited pediatric research in this area, these hypotheses may still be useful to help guide the design and interpretation of studies in pediatric populations. The literature indicates that a certain level of task engagement is required for a task to be sensitive to sleep restriction. Performance on tasks that meet but do not exceed this level are vulnerable to impairments due to decreased vigilance. Additionally, tasks that meet the necessary level of task engagement and require the greatest PFC involvement are likely the most vulnerable.

SUMMARY

Children are not getting the amounts of sleep recommended for different age groups, although these recommendations are based more on expert opinion than on empirical results. Experimental evidence is now available, however, demonstrating that reduced durations of sleep impair several aspects of cognitive and emotional functioning in otherwise typically developing children. The high prevalence of either short sleep or sleep disorders among children and the multitude of negative consequences make it especially concerning that society does not place more value on sleep. To reduce the incidence of inadequate sleep and its resulting negative effects, it is important to improve awareness of developmentally appropriate sleep and healthy sleep habits.

Educating children, parents, and professionals on the topic of sleep should involve encouragement of healthy sleep habits and discouragement of unhealthy sleep habits. The literature has repeatedly demonstrated that the use of electronic technologies prior to bedtime, the presence of electronic devices in the bedroom, and caffeine intake have serious negative consequences for sleep quality and quantity. Thus, it is concerning that approximately 50% of school-aged children have televisions in their bedrooms and more than 40% of school-aged children consume at least 1 caffeinated beverage daily.[53] E-mail and texting are undoubtedly further eating into usual sleep hours for many children.

Positive aspects of sleep practices, such as having a consistent bedtime routine, are related to longer sleep durations and better sleep quality.[53] As children move toward adolescence, there are increasing biological and psychosocial

influences that interfere with sleep,[7] which are likely to further contribute to sleep problems. Thus, targeting children prior to adolescence and instilling healthy sleep habits at that stage are likely to be beneficial approaches, which may be best initiated through the education system.[30]

Education should lead to increased awareness and recognition of sleep problems. Early identification of problems can lead to effective treatment resulting in improved daytime functioning. It is critical that parents and health care providers routinely discuss sleep issues with families and that children be screened regularly for potential sleep problems, in particular children who have problems with emotional regulation or cognitive functioning.

REFERENCES

1. Carskadon MA, Harvey K, William CD. Sleep loss in young adolescents. Sleep 1981;4(3):312.
2. Fallone G, Acebo C, Arnedt JT, et al. Effects of acute sleep restriction on behavior, sustained attention, and response inhibition in children. Percept Mot Skills 2001;93(1):213–29.
3. Wolfson AR, Carskadon MA. Sleep schedules and daytime functioning in adolescents. Child Dev 1998;69(4):875.
4. Wahlstrom K. Changing times: findings from the first longitudinal study of later high school start times. NASSP Bull 2002;86(633):3–21.
5. Sadeh A, Gruber R, Raviv A. The effects of sleep restriction and extension on school-age children: what a difference an hour makes. Child Dev 2003;74(2): 444–55.
6. Randazzo AC, Muehlbach MJ, Schweitzer PK, et al. Cognitive function following acute sleep restriction in children ages 10–14. Sleep 1998;21(8):861–8.
7. Dahl RE, Harvey AG. Sleep in children and adolescents with behavioral and emotional disorders. Sleep Med Clin 2007;2(3):501–11.
8. Alfano CA, Beidel DC, Turner SM, et al. Preliminary evidence for sleep complaints among children referred for anxiety. Sleep Med 2006;7:467–73.
9. Hudson JL, Gradisar M, Gamble A, et al. The sleep patterns and problems of clinically anxious children. Behav Res Ther 2009;47:339–44.
10. Paavonen EJ, Almqvist F, Tamminen T, et al. Poor sleep and psychiatric symptoms at school: an epidemiological study. Eur Child Adolesc Psychiatry 2002;11(1):10–7.
11. Smaldone A, Honig JC, Byrne MW. Does assessing sleep inadequacy across its continuum inform associations with child and family health? J Pediatr Health Care 2009;23(6):394–404.
12. Johnson EO, Roth T, Breslau N. The association of insomnia with anxiety disorders and

depression: exploration of the direction of risk. J Psychiatr Res 2006;40(8):700–8.

13. Bertocci MA, Dahl RE, Williamson DE, et al. Subjective sleep complaints in pediatric depression: a controlled study and comparison with EEG measures of sleep and waking. J Am Acad Child Adolesc Psychiatry 2005;44(11):1158–66.

14. Forbes EE, Bertocci MA, Gregory AM, et al. Objective sleep in pediatric anxiety disorders and major depressive disorder. J Am Acad Child Adolesc Psychiatry 2008;47(2):148–55.

15. Rapoport J, Elkins R, Langer DH, et al. Childhood obsessive-compulsive disorder. Am J Psychiatry 1981;138(12):1545–54.

16. Sadeh A, McGuire JP, Sachs H, et al. Sleep and psychological characteristics of children on a psychiatric inpatient unit. J Am Acad Child Adolesc Psychiatry 1995;34(6):813–9.

17. Gregory AM, Van der Ende J, Willis TA, et al. Parent-reported sleep problems during development and self-reported anxiety/depression, attention problems, and aggressive behavior later in life. Arch Pediatr Adolesc Med 2008;162:330–5 (1538–3628).

18. Fredriksen K, Rhodes J, Reddy R, et al. Sleepless in Chicago: tracking the effects of adolescent sleep loss during the middle school years. Child Dev 2004;75(1):84–95.

19. Aronen ET, Paavonen EJ, Fjallberg M, et al. Sleep and psychiatric symptoms in school-age children. J Am Acad Child Adolesc Psychiatry 2000;39(4):502–8.

20. Vriend JL, Davidson FD, Corkum PV, et al. Sleep quantity and quality in relation to daytime functioning in children. Child Health Care 2012; 41(3):204–22.

21. Talbot LS, McGlinchey EL, Kaplan KA, et al. Sleep deprivation in adolescents and adults: changes in affect. Emotion 2010;10:831–41.

22. Vriend JL, Davidson F, Corkum PV, et al. Altering sleep duration affects emotional functioning, memory, and attention in children. J Pediatr Psychol 2013;38(10):1058–69.

23. Epstein R, Chillag N, Lavie P. Starting time of school: effects on daytime functioning of fifth-grade children in Israel. Sleep 1998;21(3):250–6.

24. Weissbluth M, Davis AT, Poncher J, et al. Signs of airway obstruction during sleep and behavioral, developmental, and academic problems. J Dev Behav Pediatr 1983;4(2):119–21.

25. Könen T, Dirk J, Schmiedek F. Cognitive benefits of last night's sleep: daily variations in children's sleep behavior are related to working memory fluctuations. J Child Psychol Psychiatry 2015;56:171–82.

26. Sadeh A, Gruber R, Raviv A. Sleep, neurobehavioral functioning, and behavior problems in school-age children. Child Dev 2002;73(2):405–17.

27. Gruber R, Grizenko N, Schwartz G, et al. Performance on the continuous performance test in children with ADHD is associated with sleep efficiency. Sleep 2007;30(8):1003–9.

28. Steenari M, Vuontela V, Paavonen EJ, et al. Working memory and sleep in 6- to 13-year-old schoolchildren. J Am Acad Child Adolesc Psychiatry 2003; 42(1):85–92.

29. Fallone G, Acebo C, Seifer R, et al. Experimental restriction of sleep opportunity in children: effects on teacher ratings. Sleep 2005;28(12):1561–7.

30. Gruber R, Wiebe S, Montecalvo L, et al. Impact of sleep restriction on neurobehavioral functioning of children with attention deficit hyperactivity disorder. Sleep 2011;34(3):315–23.

31. Peters JD, Biggs SN, Bauer KM, et al. The sensitivity of a PDA-based psychomotor vigilance task to sleep restriction in 10-year-old girls. J Sleep Res 2009; 18(2):173–7.

32. Gruber R, Laviolette R, Deluca P, et al. Short sleep duration is associated with poor performance on IQ measures in healthy school-age children. Sleep Med 2010;11(3):289–94.

33. Carskadon M, Harvey K, Dement WC. Acute restriction of nocturnal sleep in children. Percept Mot Skills 1981;53(1):103–12.

34. Beebe D, Fallone G, Godiwala N, et al. Feasibility and behavioral effects of an at-home multi-night sleep restriction protocol for adolescents. J Child Psychol Psychiatry 2008;49(9):915–23.

35. Beebe DW, Rose D, Amin R. Attention, learning, and arousal of experimentally sleep-restricted adolescents in a simulated classroom. J Adolesc Health 2010;47(5):523–5.

36. Beebe D, Difrancesco MW, Tlustos SJ, et al. Preliminary fMRI findings in experimentally sleep-restricted adolescents engaged in a working memory task. Behav Brain Funct 2009;5:9.

37. Walker MP. Sleep-dependent memory processing. Harv Rev Psychiatry 2008;16(5):287–98.

38. Lim J, Dinges DF. A meta-analysis of the impact of short-term sleep deprivation on cognitive variables. Psychol Bull 2010;136(3):375–89.

39. Killgore WD. Effects of sleep deprivation on cognition. Prog Brain Res 2010;185:105–29.

40. Balkin TJ, Rupp T, Picchioni D, et al. Sleep loss and sleepiness: current issues. Chest 2008;134(3):653–60.

41. Minkel J, Htaik O, Banks S, et al. Emotional expressiveness in sleep-deprived healthy adults. Behav Sleep Med 2011;9(1):5–14.

42. Zohar D, Tzischinsky O, Epstein R, et al. The effects of sleep loss on medical residents' emotional reactions to work events: a cognitive-energy model. Sleep 2005;28(1):47–54.

43. Harrison Y, Horne JA. The impact of sleep deprivation on decision making: a review. J Exp Psychol Appl 2000;6(3):236–49.

44. Franzen PL, Siegle GJ, Buysse DJ. Relationships between affect, vigilance, and sleepiness following sleep deprivation. J Sleep Res 2008;17(1):34–41.

45. Davidson RJ, Lewis DA, Alloy LB, et al. Neural and behavioral substrates of mood and mood regulation. Biol Psychiatry 2002;52(6):478–502.

46. Hariri AR, Bookheimer SY, Mazziotta JC. Modulating emotional responses: effects of a neocortical network on the limbic system. Neuroreport 2000; 11(1):43–8.

47. Urry HL, van Reekum CM, Johnstone T, et al. Amygdala and ventromedial prefrontal cortex are inversely coupled during regulation of negative affect and predict the diurnal pattern of cortisol secretion among older adults. J Neurosci 2006; 26(16):4415–25.

48. Sterpenich V, Albouy G, Bloy M, et al. Sleep-related hippocampo-cortical interplay during emotional memory recollection. PLoS Biol 2007;5(11):282.

49. Yoo S, Hu PT, Gujar N, et al. A deficit in the ability to form new human memories without sleep. Nat Neurosci 2007;10(3):385–92.

50. Magill RA, Waters WF, Bray GA, et al. Effects of tyrosine, phentermine, caffeine D-amphetamine, and placebo on cognitive and motor deficits during sleep deprivation. Nutr Neurosci 2003;6(4):237–46.

51. Smith AP, Maben A. Effects of sleep deprivation, lunch, and personality on performance, mood, and cardiovascular function. Physiol Behav 1993;54(5): 967–72.

52. Pilcher JJ, Band D, Odle-Dusseau H, et al. Human performance under sustained operations and acute sleep deprivation conditions: toward a model of controlled attention. Aviat Space Environ Med 2007;78(5):B15–24.

53. Mindell JA, Meltzer LJ, Carskadon MA, et al. Developmental aspects of sleep hygiene: findings from the 2004 National Sleep Foundation Sleep in America poll. Sleep Med 2009;10(7):771–9.

The Relations Between Sleep, Personality, Behavioral Problems, and School Performance in Adolescents

Ralph E. Schmidt, PhD[a,b,*], Martial Van der Linden, PhD[a,b]

KEYWORDS

- Adolescence • Emotion regulation • Personality • School performance • Sleep

KEY POINTS

- Adolescents on average do not get the recommended amount of more than 9 hours of sleep per night.
- Delaying school start times allows adolescents to get more sleep, thereby increasing attendance rates and academic achievement, especially in evening-type individuals.
- Neuroticism, anxiety, type D personality, perfectionism, and impulsivity are risk factors for sleep problems.
- Insufficient sleep in adolescents contributes to problems with emotional-behavioral regulation and, as a consequence, to a range of potentially self-harming and other-harming behaviors, such as drug use, risky driving, hyperactivity, and aggression.
- Insufficient sleep in adolescents also contributes to poor academic achievement.
- The negative effects of insufficient sleep on emotional-behavioral regulation and academic achievement are more pronounced in adolescents from families with lower socioeconomic status.
- Multicomponent treatment programs specifically designed for adolescents have been developed on the basis of cognitive-behavioral therapy for insomnia.

SLEEP NEEDS AND PATTERNS IN ADOLESCENTS

Accumulating empirical evidence suggests that, across different countries and cultures, adolescents do not get the recommended amount of sleep. Although longitudinal studies of sleep needs through puberty have suggested that adolescents require more than 9.0 hours of sleep at night, on average they obtain between 7.5 and 8.5 hours per night, with approximately 25% of adolescents obtaining fewer than 6.5 hours and only approximately 15% obtaining 8.5 hours or more.[1] As for gender differences, a meta-analysis has indicated that, on school days, girls sleep on average 11 minutes per night more than do boys, and that on nonschool days, girls sleep 29 minutes more.[2] Across adolescence, sleep time declines on average by 14 minutes per year of age on

[a] Department of Psychology, Swiss Center for Affective Sciences, University of Geneva, Chemin des Mines 9, Geneva CH-1202, Switzerland; [b] Cognitive Psychopathology and Neuropsychology Unit, Department of Psychology, University of Geneva, Boulevard du Pont d'Arve 40, Geneva CH-1205, Switzerland
* Corresponding author. Department of Psychology, University of Geneva, Boulevard du Pont d'Arve 40, Geneva CH-1205, Switzerland.
E-mail address: Ralph.Schmidt@unige.ch

Sleep Med Clin 10 (2015) 117–123
http://dx.doi.org/10.1016/j.jsmc.2015.02.007
1556-407X/15/$ – see front matter © 2015 Elsevier Inc. All rights reserved.

school days and by 7 minutes per year of age on nonschool days, essentially due to a shift toward later bedtimes.[2,3] On nonschool days, adolescents typically sleep 1.5 hours longer than they do on school days, suggesting that they accrue a sleep debt across the week that is relieved by oversleep on weekends.[3]

Regarding cultural differences, 2 meta-analyses have found that adolescents from Asian countries sleep significantly less each night than do adolescents from North America, Australia, and Europe, essentially because of later bedtimes.[2,3] Another recent comprehensive meta-analysis of data on 690,747 children and adolescents from 20 countries has revealed that between 1905 and 2008, sleep duration generally decreased by more than 1 hour per night. However, rates of change varied according to geographic region: whereas sleep duration decreased in Europe (not including Scandinavia and the United Kingdom), the United States, Canada, and Asia, it increased in Scandinavia, the United Kingdom, and Australia.[4]

Apart from intrinsic factors, such as the pubertal shift in chronotype preference from morningness to eveningness[5] or specific sleep disorders (eg, insomnia, obstructive sleep apnea, restless legs syndrome), a number of extrinsic factors may contribute to insufficient sleep in teens; namely, extracurricular activities, after-school jobs, and homework.[1] For instance, nearly 20% of a sample of high school students indicated spending 20 hours per week or more on extracurricular activities (eg, sports, music, social clubs) and those students also reported significantly later bedtimes and less total sleep time when compared with students who spent fewer than 20 hours in extracurricular activities.[6] Moreover, almost 60% of this sample of high school students reported having a part-time job and nearly 30% indicated working more than 20 hours per week. As with extracurricular activities, students who worked more than 20 hours per week at a part-time job indicated significantly later bedtimes and less total sleep time when compared with students who worked less than 20 hours per week.[6] Engaging in extracurricular activities or holding a job also may delay school homework completion, thereby further postponing bedtime.[1]

When at home in the evening, adolescents increasingly use electronic devices for information, communication, and entertainment, whereby sleep also may be delayed.[7] In the hour before going to bed on school nights, 76% of adolescents report watching TV, 44% surfing the Internet or sending instant messages, 40% talking on the phone, and 26% playing electronic or video games.[8] A review of 36 studies with school-aged children and adolescents showed that electronic media use is significantly related to delayed bedtime and shorter total sleep time.[9] Several mechanisms may mediate the effect of electronic media use on sleep: (1) media use may directly displace sleep or other activities related to good sleep hygiene (eg, physical activity); (2) media use may increase sleep-interfering physiologic, affective, and cognitive arousal; and (3) bright light exposure from television and computer screens may delay melatonin secretion, thereby delaying the circadian rhythm.[9] As might be expected, adolescents reaching pathologic levels of electronic media use run a particularly high risk of suffering from sleep problems.[10]

After going to bed late in the evening because of extracurricular activities, jobs, school homework, or use of electronic devices, adolescents typically have to get up early in the morning to attend school, resulting in insufficient sleep. A number of observational and intervention studies have consistently shown that when school start times are delayed by 25 to 85 minutes, bedtimes typically do not change and adolescents get on average 30 to 60 minutes more sleep.[11–15] In turn, this additional sleep time is associated with higher attendance rates, less sleepiness and dozing in class, lower depression scores, reduced caffeine consumption, better concentration, and higher grades.[11–15]

PERSONALITY TRAITS AS RISK FACTORS FOR SLEEP PROBLEMS IN ADOLESCENTS

It has been postulated that a number of personality traits might make adolescents and adults vulnerable to developing sleep problems, particularly when under stress.[16] Early research indicated that internalization, or the excessive inhibition of outward behaviors, might entail a state of constant emotional arousal, thereby contributing to sleep disturbance. Accumulating evidence does indeed suggest that poor sleepers often display high scores on internalization, neuroticism (= enduring tendency to experience negative emotional states), anxiety, and perfectionism.[16] In a recent extension of this line of research, it has been found that adolescents with a type D personality, or distressed personality (= tendency to experience negative emotions and, concomitantly, to inhibit self-expression in social interaction), incur an approximately 4 times higher risk of having sleep disturbances.[17] The recent literature also suggests that the relations between personality traits and sleep problems are best conceptualized as bidirectional. For instance, a longitudinal study has shown that sleep-onset problems during adolescence are a direct risk factor for heightened neuroticism in midlife.[18]

Another line of research has revealed that not only excessive inhibition of behaviors, as in internalization, but also excessive disinhibition of behaviors, as in externalization, may result in an affective imbalance that manifests itself in sleep-interfering emotional arousal. For example, studies with undergraduate students have shown that those scoring high on impulsive urgency are particularly prone to experience feelings of regret, shame, and guilt at bedtime, likely because they compare their rash daytime behavior with how they would have liked to behave.[19] Impulsive urgency can be defined as the tendency to act rashly, especially under conditions of negative affect,[20] and has been associated with the use of inappropriate emotion-regulation strategies, such as self-attacking and rumination, which may contribute to sleep-interfering mental activity at bedtime.[21,22]

Finally, the personality dimension of chronotype preference (morningness/eveningness; "larks" vs "owls") is of importance when considering the relations among sleep, daytime behavior, and school performance in adolescents. Self-report studies have associated eveningness with later bedtimes, shorter sleep, and reduced sleep quality on school nights, greater tendency to fall asleep at school, diminished alertness, depressed mood, and poorer school performance.[23,24] An experimental study in which intelligence tests were administered to adolescents at their optimal and nonoptimal times of day lent further support to the findings from the self-report studies.[25] Specifically, a 6-point difference in IQ estimates was observed as a function of the match between the individual's circadian arousal pattern and the time of testing. Moreover, evening-type adolescents obtained higher scores on measures of attention problems and aggressive behavior, suggesting that they have comparatively more conduct problems at home and school.

SLEEP AND BEHAVIORAL PROBLEMS IN ADOLESCENTS

Independently of circadian phase preference, insufficient sleep in adolescents has been associated with a number of potentially self-harming or other-harming behaviors, such as cigarette smoking, alcohol consumption, drug use, and risky sexual behaviors.[26–29] In addition, more than half of 10th to 12th graders report drowsy driving in the past year,[5] which is all the more worrying because motor vehicle accidents account for the greatest number of adolescent deaths in the United States.[1]

Longitudinal investigations have, furthermore, associated insufficient sleep with a range of externalizing behaviors, such as hyperactivity, irritability, aggression, and other conduct problems.[30] These associations also were highlighted by an intervention study that examined the effects of a 6-week behavioral sleep treatment in adolescents with substance-related difficulties.[31] It was found that increases in sleep time were associated with decreases in aggressive ideation and aggressive actions occurring during conflicts. These findings in adolescents indicate that inadequate sleep undermines emotional and behavioral regulation,[32] in accord with sleep deprivation studies in adults, which suggest that sleep loss impairs the functional connectivity between the prefrontal cortex (area involved in voluntary control) and the amygdala (area involved in emotional reactions).[33]

Some longitudinal studies have indicated that the negative effects of inadequate sleep on behavioral adjustment are particularly marked in adolescents from homes of lower socioeconomic status (SES).[32] Other longitudinal studies have suggested that the initial presence of sleep problems is less important in predicting later behavioral adjustment than whether these problems persist or worsen over time.[34]

SLEEP AND SCHOOL PERFORMANCE IN ADOLESCENTS

Since the 1980s, a series of studies have strongly suggested that self-reported short sleep duration, poor sleep quality, late bed and rise times, and irregular sleep schedules are negatively associated with academic performance for adolescents from middle school through the college years.[22,35] A meta-analytic review of one longitudinal and 16 cross-sectional studies found that sleep duration, sleep quality, and sleepiness were all negatively related to school performance in children and adolescents.[36] The effect was strongest for sleepiness, followed by sleep quality and sleep duration. Moreover, the effect sizes were larger for younger participants, which might, according to the investigators of the study, be explained by the important maturation-related changes of the prefrontal cortex in early adolescence.

Few longitudinal investigations have been done, however, on the effects of chronic short sleep on scholastic performance in adolescents. One such study has recently found that late school year bedtime was associated with worse educational outcomes and emotional distress 6 to 8 years later, but that short total sleep time was not longitudinally related to these outcomes.[37] As the investigators of this study note, in accord with the findings of the earlier-mentioned meta-analysis,[36] the effects of short sleep might be most pronounced in young adolescents because with maturation, older adolescents may experience a decrease in sensitivity to sleep loss and extended wakefulness.[38,39] Moreover, again in line with the findings of the meta-analysis,[36] another recent study suggests that sleepiness may be a better predictor of objective school performance than either sleep quality or sleep duration.[40] According to the investigators of this study, sleepiness during the first hours of school may be a key mechanism whereby insufficient sleep negatively impacts academic performance.

Emerging research also suggests that lower SES is related to shorter sleep duration and that, in addition, the negative effects of inadequate sleep on academic achievement may be comparatively greater in children and adolescents from lower SES families.[32] Among the various indicators of SES, the level of parental education turned out to be an important moderator between sleep and scholastic performance in children and adolescents. Parental education presumably is a proxy for a wide range of circumstances and conditions that can amplify or dampen the effects of insufficient sleep. For instance, lower educational level may be linked to more family stressors or less parental monitoring. In combination with such factors, insufficient sleep may contribute to the so-called achievement gap; that is, academic underachievement in children and adolescents from lower SES families.[32]

The exact mechanisms whereby sleep may affect academic achievement still remain to be explored. The available empirical evidence indicates that academic performance results from a complex interplay among multiple factors, including cognitive functioning, achievement motivation, personality, and emotional-behavioral regulation.[32,41] As for cognitive functioning, correlational studies and experimental investigations suggest that inadequate sleep leads to more daytime sleepiness, inattention, and impairments in executive functioning, which may all adversely affect academic achievement in children and adolescents.[34,41] Executive functioning refers to higher-order, prefrontal cortex–related cognitive processes, including impulse control, set shifting, and working memory, which underlie the monitoring and control of thought and action. Longitudinal studies have revealed that sleep problems in childhood, especially if they persist, may predict executive functioning in later childhood and adolescence.[42,43] Importantly, experimental evidence also indicates that even very

moderate (eg, "just 1 more TV show" of 1 hour), but accumulated, sleep loss may impair executive functioning in children and adolescents.[41] Of note is a consistent body of experimental evidence from studies with adults suggesting that sleep is essential for processes of memory consolidation[44]; processes that are also pivotal for academic performance in adolescents.[45]

Academic success also depends on emotional-behavioral regulation, in particular the ability and motivation to behave in compliance with teachers' expectations within the constraints of a typical school environment and to avoid conflict with teachers and classmates.[32] Recent evidence suggests that certain personality traits may predispose adolescents toward emotional-behavioral dysregulation, thereby increasing the risk of poor academic performance. For instance, one longitudinal study found that adolescents scoring high on impulsive urgency were particularly prone to report symptoms of insomnia, signs of hyperactivity, and poor school grades, with hyperactivity partially mediating the negative effect of sleep problems on school grades.[46] Highlighting the role of motivation, another study found that chronic sleep reduction in preadolescents was linked to lower achievement motivation, a poorer self-view as a pupil, and a more negative perception of the teacher's behavior, and that these 3 variables partially mediated the relation between chronic sleep reduction and lower school achievement.[47]

INTERVENTIONS FOR SLEEP PROBLEMS IN ADOLESCENTS

Over the past years, several researchers have begun to develop sleep intervention programs that are specifically adapted to children and adolescents. For instance, a comprehensive sleep treatment for youth has been proposed that encompasses the following components[48]: (1) assisting the young person to find his or her internal motivation for enhancing sleep; (2) providing sleep and circadian education to correct unhelpful sleep habits while constructing new healthy sleep habits; (3) practicing "stimulus control," that is, limiting sleep-incompatible behaviors within the bedroom environment (eg, television watching or text messaging), while increasing cues for sleep-compatible behaviors; (4) addressing worry and rumination, for example by diary writing or scheduling a "worry period" to encourage the processing of worry several hours before bedtime; (5) targeting media use and social activities to achieve an earlier bedtime; and (6) preventing relapse by summarizing the young person's learning and achievements, as well as by setting specific goals and goal-conducive plans for the future.

A recent randomized controlled trial of cognitive-behavioral therapy (CBT) for children aged 7 to 13 found that compared with waitlist controls, children receiving CBT showed significant improvements in sleep latency, wake after sleep onset, and sleep efficiency, with all gains being maintained 6 months posttreatment.[49] In another recent study, a school-based intervention aimed to provide adolescents with information about sleep and to motivate them to make changes in several target sleep behaviors.[50] Although the intervention successfully enhanced adolescents' knowledge about sleep and their motivation to regularize out-of-bed times, parallel improvements in sleep and daytime functioning were not significantly different from the control group. A general problem with school-based sleep-promoting programs is that they effectively enhance sleep knowledge but usually do not succeed in maintaining sleep behavior changes.[51] This shortcoming highlights the importance of integrating motivational components into the programs; for example, motivational interviewing in an individually tailored setting.[51]

Regarding possible interventions at the organizational level of schools, research has revealed that setting later start times leads to more sleep in adolescents, as mentioned earlier. Moreover, given that adolescents from lower SES families are particularly at risk of getting insufficient sleep and suffering from the negative consequences on academic achievement, individual, group, and school-level interventions to improve sleep in this group of adolescents merit special attention by researchers and practitioners.

SUMMARY

Empirical evidence suggests that, across different countries and cultures, adolescents do not get the recommended amount of at least 9 hours of sleep per night. The scientific literature has identified a number of factors that are liable to postpone bedtime in adolescents and in this way to contribute to insufficient sleep; namely, extracurricular activities, after-school jobs, homework, and electronic media use (eg, TV, computer, smartphone) in the evening. At the same time, research indicates that insufficient sleep in adolescents contributes to problems with emotional-behavioral regulation and, as a consequence, to a range of potentially self-harming and other-harming behaviors, such as drug use, risky driving, hyperactivity, and aggression. Moreover, insufficient sleep may impair academic achievement, especially in adolescents from lower SES families, and several personality traits may render individuals particularly vulnerable to insufficient sleep and its negative consequences; for example, neuroticism, impulsivity, or eveningness. Regarding sleep-promoting interventions, delaying school start times allows adolescents to get more sleep, whereby attendance rates, attention, and academic achievement are increased, especially in evening-type individuals. In addition, multicomponent treatment programs are available that have been developed on the basis of CBT for insomnia and specifically adapted for use with adolescents.

REFERENCES

1. Moore M, Meltzer LJ. The sleepy adolescent: causes and consequences of sleepiness in teens. Paediatr Respir Rev 2008;9:114–21.
2. Olds T, Blunden S, Petkov J, et al. The relationships between sex, age, geography and time in bed in adolescents: a meta-analysis of data from 23 countries. Sleep Med Rev 2010;14:371–8.
3. Gradisar M, Gardner G, Dohnt H. Recent worldwide sleep patterns and problems during adolescence: a review and meta-analysis of age, region, and sleep. Sleep Med 2011;12:110–8.
4. Matricciani L, Olds T, Petkov J. In search of lost sleep: secular trends in the sleep time of school-aged children and adolescents. Sleep Med Rev 2012;16:203–11.
5. Carskadon MA, Acebo C, Jenni OG. Regulation of adolescent sleep: implications for behavior. Ann N Y Acad Sci 2004;1021:276–91.
6. Carskadon MA. Adolescent sleepiness: increased risk in a high-risk population. Alcohol Drugs Driving 1990;6:317–28.
7. Knutson KL, Lauderdale DS. Sociodemographic and behavioral predictors of bed time and wake time among US adolescents aged 15 to 17 years. J Pediatr 2009;154:426–30.
8. National Sleep Foundation. Sleep in America Poll 2006. Available at: www.sleepfoundation.org. Accessed March 4, 2015.
9. Cain N, Gradisar M. Electronic media use and sleep in school-aged children and adolescents: a review. Sleep Med 2010;11:735–42.
10. King DL, Delfabbro PH, Zwaans T, et al. Sleep interference effects of pathological electronic media use during adolescence. Int J Ment Health Addict 2014; 12:21–35.
11. Epstein R, Chillag N, Lavie P. Starting times of school: effects of daytime functioning of fifth-grade children in Israel. Sleep 1998;21:250–6.
12. Wahistrom K. Changing times: findings from the first longitudinal study of later high school start times. NASSP Bull 2002;86:3–21.

13. Wolfson AR, Spaulding NL, Dandrow C, et al. Middle school start times: the importance of a good night's sleep for young adolescents. Behav Sleep Med 2007;5:194–209.

14. Owens JA, Belon K, Moss P. Impact of delaying school start time on adolescent sleep, mood, and behavior. Arch Pediatr Adolesc Med 2010;164: 608–13.

15. Boergers J, Gable CJ, Owens JA. Later school start time is associated with improved sleep and daytime functioning in adolescents. J Dev Behav Pediatr 2014;35:11–7.

16. Van de Laar M, Verbeek I, Pevernagie D, et al. The role of personality traits in insomnia. Sleep Med Rev 2010;14:61–8.

17. Condén E, Ekselius L, Åslund C. Type D personality is associated with sleep problems in adolescents: results from a population-based cohort study of Swedish adolescents. J Psychosom Res 2013;74: 290–5.

18. Danielsson NS, Jansson-Fröjmark M, Linton SJ, et al. Neuroticism and sleep-onset: what is the long-term connection? Pers Individ Dif 2010;48: 463–8.

19. Schmidt RE, Van der Linden M. The aftermath of rash action: sleep-interfering counterfactual thoughts and emotions. Emotion 2009;9:549–53.

20. Whiteside SP, Lynam DR. The five factor model and impulsivity: using a structural model of personality to understand impulsivity. Pers Individ Dif 2001;30: 669–89.

21. Schmidt RE, Gay P, Ghisletta P, et al. Linking impulsivity to dysfunctional thought control and insomnia: a structural equation model. J Sleep Res 2010;19:3–11.

22. Schmidt RE, Harvey AG, Van der Linden M. Cognitive and affective control in insomnia. Front Psychol 2011;22:349.

23. Wolfson AR, Carskadon MA. Understanding adolescents' sleep patterns and school performance: a critical appraisal. Sleep Med Rev 2003;7:491–506.

24. Short MA, Gradisar M, Lack LC, et al. The impact of sleep on adolescent depressed mood, alertness and academic performance. J Adolesc 2013;36: 1025–33.

25. Goldstein D, Hahn CS, Hasher L, et al. Time of day, intellectual performance, and behavioural problems in morning versus evening type adolescents: is there a synchrony effect? Pers Individ Dif 2007;41: 431–40.

26. Johnson EO, Breslau N. Sleep problems and substance use in adolescents. Drug Alcohol Depend 2001;64:1–17.

27. Wong MM, Brower KJ, Fitzgerald HE, et al. Sleep problems in early childhood and early onset of alcohol and other drug use in adolescence. Alcohol Clin Exp Res 2004;28:578–87.

28. O'Brien EM, Mindell JA. Sleep and risk-taking behavior in adolescents. Behav Sleep Med 2005;3: 113–33.

29. Shochat T, Cohen-Zion M, Tzischinsky O. Functional consequences of inadequate sleep in adolescents: a systematic review. Sleep Med Rev 2014;18:75–87.

30. Gregory AM, Eley TC, O'Connor TG, et al. Etiologies of associations between childhood sleep problems and behavioral problems in a large twin sample. J Am Acad Child Adolesc Psychiatry 2004;43: 744–51.

31. Haynes PL, Bootzin RR, Smith L, et al. Sleep and aggression in substance-abusing adolescents: results from an integrative behavioral sleep-treatment program. Sleep 2006;29:512–20.

32. Buckhalt JA. Insufficient sleep and the socioeconomic status achievement gap. Child Dev Perspect 2011;5:59–65.

33. Yoo SS, Gujar N, Hu P, et al. The human emotional brain without sleep—a prefrontal amygdala disconnect. Curr Biol 2007;17:877–8.

34. Beebe DW. Cognitive, behavioral, and functional consequences of inadequate sleep in children and adolescents. Pediatr Clin North Am 2011;58:649–65.

35. Curcio G, Ferrara M, De Gennaro L. Sleep loss, learning capacity and academic performance. Sleep Med Rev 2006;10:323–37.

36. Dewald JF, Meijer AM, Oort FJ, et al. The influence of sleep quality, sleep duration and sleepiness on school performance in children and adolescents: a meta-analytic review. Sleep Med Rev 2010;14: 179–89.

37. Asarnow LD, McGlinchey E, Harvey AG. The effects of bedtime and sleep duration on academic and emotional outcomes in a nationally representative sample of adolescents. J Adolesc Health 2014;54: 350–6.

38. Jenni OG, Achermann P, Carskadon MA. Homeostatic sleep regulation in adolescents. Sleep 2005; 28:1446–54.

39. Taylor DJ, Jenni OG, Acebo C, et al. Sleep tendency during extended wakefulness: insights into adolescent sleep regulation and behavior. J Sleep Res 2005;14:239–44.

40. Boschloo A, Krabbendam L, Dekker S, et al. Subjective sleepiness and sleep quality in adolescents are related to objective and subjective measures of school performance. Front Psychol 2013;4:38.

41. Sadeh A. Consequences of sleep loss or sleep disruption in children. Sleep Med Clin 2007;2:513–20.

42. Friedman NP, Corley RP, Hewitt JK, et al. Individual differences in childhood sleep problems predict later cognitive executive control. Sleep 2009;32:323–33.

43. Bernier A, Carlson SM, Bordeleau S, et al. Relations between physiological and cognitive regulatory systems: infant sleep regulation and subsequent executive functioning. Child Dev 2010;81:1739–52.

44. Stickgold R, Walker MP. Sleep-dependent memory consolidation and re-consolidation. Sleep Med 2007;8:331–43.

45. Carskadon MA. Sleep's effects on cognition and learning in adolescence. Prog Brain Res 2011;190: 137–43.

46. Schmidt RE, Gomez J, Gay P, et al. A longitudinal investigation into the relations between personality, sleep, conduct problems, and school performance in adolescents. Sleep 2009;32:A81.

47. Meijer AM. Chronic sleep reduction, functioning at school and school achievement in preadolescents. J Sleep Res 2008;17:395–405.

48. Dahl RE, Harvey AG. Sleep in children and adolescents with behavioral and emotional disorders. Sleep Med Clin 2007;2:501–11.

49. Paine S, Gradisar M. A randomised controlled trial of cognitive-behaviour therapy for behavioural insomnia of childhood in school-aged children. Behav Res Ther 2011;49:379–88.

50. Cain N, Gradisar M, Moseley L. A motivational school-based intervention for adolescent sleep problems. Sleep Med 2011;12:246–51.

51. Cassoff J, Knäuper B, Michaelsen S, et al. School-based sleep promotion programs: effectiveness, feasibility and insights for future research. Sleep Med Rev 2013;17:207–14.

Anxiety Disorders and Sleep in Children and Adolescents

Thomas A. Willis, BSc, PhD[a], Alice M. Gregory, BA, PhD[b],*

KEYWORDS

- Adolescent • Anxiety • Bidirectionality • Child • Internalizing • Sleep

KEY POINTS

- There seems to be a robust association between sleep and anxiety in children and adolescents.
- Evidence comes from cross-sectional and longitudinal studies, and community and clinical samples.
- Variation in the definitions and measurement methods used need to be considered when interpreting results.
- Potential mechanisms suggested include physiologic and psychological processes.

INTRODUCTION

Sleep problems are common in youth, with approximately 40% of children aged 4 to 11 years experiencing difficulties for at least brief periods.[1] In clinically anxious children, this proportion seems to be substantially higher. Alfano and colleagues[2] reported that 85% of a sample of anxiety-disordered 7 to 14 year olds had clinically significant sleep disturbance scores.

There are good reasons to focus on youth when considering the association between sleep difficulties and anxiety. First, it is known that disorders in adults typically begin early in life. For example, in anxiety-disordered adults, a substantial proportion (38%) was diagnosed with anxiety by age 15 years.[3] Second, many studies have identified that the two problems frequently co-occur in pediatric populations.[4] Third, a growing body of research has examined the directionality of the relationship, particularly the possibility that disturbed sleep in childhood may predict anxiety later in life.[5] If it is the case that sleep disturbance acts as an early risk factor for developing an anxiety disorder (or vice versa), then efforts can be made to identify those individuals at potential risk and who may benefit most from intervention.

This article considers associations between sleep disturbance and anxiety in children and adolescents. First, some important methodologic issues and inconsistencies are considered. This is followed by a summary of some key findings from the literature, from both cross-sectional and longitudinal research. A variety of potential mechanisms by which sleep and anxiety may be related have been suggested, and a selection of these are then outlined.

METHODOLOGIC ISSUES

There are some important considerations when interpreting work in this field that need to be outlined before introducing the literature: definition of sleep

Disclosure Statement: The authors have nothing to disclose.
[a] Leeds Institute of Health Sciences, University of Leeds, 101 Clarendon Road, Leeds LS2 9LJ, UK; [b] Department of Psychology, Goldsmiths, University of London, Lewisham Way, New Cross, London SE14 6NW, UK
* Corresponding author.
E-mail address: a.gregory@gold.ac.uk

Sleep Med Clin 10 (2015) 125–131
http://dx.doi.org/10.1016/j.jsmc.2015.02.002

problems, measurement of sleep, and conceptualizations of anxiety.

Definition of Sleep Problems

The term "sleep-related problems" is commonly used in research in this field[1] and can encompass a variety of issues. These may include dyssomnias, such as symptoms of insomnia, which may include difficulty falling asleep, or frequent nighttime waking. Alternatively, they may refer to parasomnias, including sleepwalking or night terrors. Moreover, some research has focused on specific symptoms, such as sleep duration or sleep onset latency (ie, time taken to fall asleep), whereas others have taken a broader perspective and considered a pool of sleep variables. For example, Gregory and O'Connor[6] investigated "total sleep problems," a heterogeneous group of sleep difficulties providing a general sense of sleep quality. Furthermore, the classification of disorders may also vary depending on the diagnostic system being used (eg, the *Diagnostic and Statistical Manual of Mental Disorders*[7] or the *International Classification of Sleep Disorders*[8]).

Measurement of Sleep

A second issue concerns the diverse range of methods used to assess sleep. For example, it is possible to use objective methods, such as actigraphy, a watch-like device that records movement and can be used to make inferences about sleep patterns, or polysomnography, often considered the gold-standard measurement technique. Furthermore, there are innovative new methods to assess sleep that may become more important in due course.[9] Largely for reasons of cost and ease of use, most studies use subjective measures of sleep, such as questionnaires or sleep diaries. Some studies use single-item measures. For instance, the children and adolescents investigated by Alfano and colleagues[2] were asked if they have trouble sleeping and/or trouble waking in the morning; or a longitudinal French cohort study where parents were asked, "Does your child have sleep problems?."[10] Others use multi-term measures.[11] Gregory and colleagues[12] compared subjective (ie, sleep items from the Child Behaviour Checklist) and objective measures (ie, actigraphy, sleep laboratory) of sleep. Although there was some evidence of correspondence between methods (eg, the Child Behavior Checklist item "trouble sleeping" was associated with sleep diary and actigraphy-assessed sleep latency), many variables showed no association. The use of subjective and objective measures of sleep is likely to offer the most comprehensive assessment of how an individual is sleeping.

A further consideration is the informant: sleep data may be provided by parents or the child/adolescent themselves. The methods used may contribute to the results observed: some studies have shown that a greater number of sleep problems are revealed using child-reported (as against parent-reported) data.[13,14] This pattern seems to be reversed in clinical samples, with parents reporting more problems than the children themselves.[2,15]

Conceptualization of Anxiety

Finally, there is similar heterogeneity in the measurement of anxiety. For example, sleep has been examined in relation to combined anxiety-depression[6,16] or the broader construct "internalizing symptoms," which includes depression and anxiety together with somatic complaints.[10] Others have focused on specific anxiety subtypes, such as obsessive-compulsive disorder (OCD), or most commonly generalized anxiety disorder (GAD).[2,15] Furthermore, as outlined later, samples may comprise community-based children and adolescents, or be drawn from clinically diagnosed anxious youth.

This article considers the results from studies that have used differing conceptualizations of sleep difficulties and anxiety, and a variety of assessment methods.

CONCURRENT ASSOCIATIONS
Sleep and Combined Anxiety/Depression

Several studies have explored the association between sleep problems and combined anxiety/depression symptomatology. This latter phenotype has been found to be associated with various aspects of disturbed sleep in nonclinical samples. For example, nightmares have been associated with emotional difficulties,[17] whereas trouble sleeping was associated with parent-reported anxiety/depression in children at age 6 years and again at age 11.[16]

Sleep and Anxiety

Many studies have explored anxiety as distinct from depression, both as a general concept and in terms of specific subtypes. Gregory and colleagues[14] investigated anxiety in relation to eight parent-reported components of sleep difficulties. Of these, bedtime resistance was associated with higher child-reported anxiety scores. However, child anxiety was not associated with the other seven aspects under consideration, including sleep onset delay and sleep duration. Others have reported a link between disturbing dreams and heightened anxiety. For example, Mindell and Barrett[18] found that anxiety rose in relation to the frequency of nightmares in a community sample of 5 to 11 year olds. In particular, the group experiencing three or more nightmares per week had parent-rated anxiety scores approaching the clinical level.

Clinical Samples

There is consistent evidence of an association between disturbed sleep and anxiety in nonclinical child and adolescent samples, but what of evidence from clinical samples? Alfano and colleagues[19] have explored these issues in clinically diagnosed anxious youth. For example, using a combination of items from parent- and clinician-rated scales, the prevalence of 'sleep-related problems' (eg, nightmares, reluctance/refusal to sleep alone) was investigated in this group. The most commonly identified problems were difficulty initiating or maintaining sleep, nightmares, and a reluctance to sleep alone. Eighty-eight percent of the sample were found to display at least one sleep-related problem, with most (55%) having at least three. A positive association was identified, whereby the number of sleep-related problems reported rose with anxiety severity. Some studies have considered the association of specific sleep problems with specific anxiety subtypes. For example, Alfano and colleagues[2] found that parasomnias were significantly more common in children with primary diagnoses of GAD or separation anxiety, than in those with social anxiety. Previous work by Alfano and colleagues also indicated that sleep problems are most closely associated with GAD and separation anxiety disorder.[19,20] It is suggested that going to bed and sleeping alone may be a more worrying event for children with diffuse anxiety or worries about separation than for those who are more troubled by particular social situations. Sleep-related problems have also been identified in children with OCD, with the total number of problems positively associated with OCD symptom severity and self-reported general anxiety.[15]

A small number of studies have used objective measures of sleep with clinical samples. For instance, Rapoport and colleagues[21] used electroencephalography to investigate the sleep of nine adolescents diagnosed with OCD. Compared with matched control subjects, those with OCD showed shortened total sleep, reduced sleep efficiency, and double the sleep latency. Similarly, Forbes and colleagues[22] used electroencephalography to assess sleep in anxiety-disordered children. Relative to

those with depression and control subjects, anxious children displayed longer sleep latency on their second night in the laboratory. In addition, the anxious group displayed more nighttime waking compared with the depressed children. More recently, Alfano and colleagues[23] used polysomnography to investigate the sleep of children diagnosed with GAD. Relative to control subjects, the children with GAD showed significantly longer sleep latency and a marginal reduction in sleep efficiency (ie, the length of time asleep relative to the total time spent in bed). However, the groups did not differ in terms of their presleep anxiety or cortisol levels.

LONGITUDINAL ASSOCIATIONS

Most studies exploring disturbed sleep and anxiety have used cross-sectional designs. Consequently, they are unable to provide information concerning the possible directionality of any associations between the two phenotypes. However, some studies have been conducted longitudinally, providing indications as to the direction of effects of the sleep disturbance–anxiety relationship. For example, Gregory and O'Connor[6] reported that sleep problems in children aged 4 years were significant predictors of combined anxiety/depression at age 13 to 15 years. However, not all studies support this relationship: Johnson and colleagues[16] reported cross-sectional associations between trouble sleeping and anxiety/depression, but found that sleep problems at 6 years were not predictive of anxiety/depression at 11 years.

A small but growing number of studies have examined the bidirectionality of the relationship (ie, whether a sleep disturbance independently predicts later anxiety, and vice versa). Generally, there is stronger evidence for the former of these pathways.[24] In the aforementioned study, Gregory and O'Connor[6] found no evidence that early anxiety/depression was predictive of later sleep problems. In a further study that looked beyond childhood, in children reported to have persistent sleep problems at 5 to 9 years, 46% proceeded to develop an anxiety disorder as an adult.[5] Jansen and colleagues[25] have attempted to explore these relationships in very young children. A large sample (N = 4782) of newborns were assessed at 2, 24, and 36 months. Dyssomnia (measured as the number of night wakings), parasomnia (the occurrence of nightmares), and short sleep duration identified at infancy or early toddlerhood were associated with a heightened risk of anxiety or depression symptoms at 3 years. The study found little evidence for the reverse relationship of anxiety or depressive symptoms preceding later sleep problems.

Recent work by Goldman-Mellor and colleagues[26] demonstrated that the presence of anxiety and internalizing symptoms during childhood (5–11 years) and/or adolescence (11–15 years) was strongly predictive of insomnia in midadulthood. This study analyzed data from a population-representative birth cohort in New Zealand (N = 1037) where participants were assessed at regular intervals, with the most recent data from age 38 years. Of note, a dose-response relationship was observed whereby the presence of anxiety diagnoses at multiple timepoints was associated with heightened risk of later insomnia. In particular, this effect was stronger when the anxiety disorder was observed during adolescence. Here, each additional anxiety diagnosis predicted a 28% increased insomnia risk. Similar results were found for depression.

However, some have demonstrated a bidirectional relationship. In a sample of more than 1000 North American children assessed between the ages of 9 and 16 years, sleep problems predicted increased GAD, whereas GAD also predicted elevated sleep problems over time.[24] Further evidence for a reciprocal relationship comes from Kelly and El-Sheikh.[27] Here, sleep disturbance at age 8 years was predictive of poorer psychological adjustment (which included anxiety, depression, and externalizing symptoms) 5 years later. To a lesser extent, adjustment also predicted changes in sleep.

POTENTIAL MECHANISMS

Further investigation to explore the pathways by which sleep and anxiety may be associated is necessary. Nevertheless, some potential mechanisms, which are not necessarily independent and are likely to interact, have been proposed. A selection of these is briefly outlined, together with possible pathways by which their effects may emerge.

Twin Studies

Twin studies typically compare the similarity of identical and nonidentical twins to draw inferences about genetic and environmental influences on traits. These studies have been informative in elucidating reasons for associations between variables (for discussion of twin studies, see[28]). A small number of twin studies of children have reported on sleep and associated traits, with one finding that parent-reported sleep disturbance in 3 year olds seemed to be genetically unrelated to all other scales assessed, including anxious behavior.[29] In contrast, common shared

environmental factors (ie, those environmental factors that act to make individuals within a family alike) seemed to influence the range of difficulties under investigation. A different picture has emerged when older youth (aged 8–16 years) were considered.[30] In particular, there did seem to be strong overlap between genetic influences on overanxious disorder and symptoms of insomnia. Although twin studies are instructive in estimating the magnitude of genetic influences on traits, they typically do not reveal much about specific genes that influence traits. This information typically comes from elsewhere (eg, association and linkage studies).

Specifying Genetic and Environmental Factors

The specific genes implicated in the overlap between various phenotypes and sleep disturbance is likely to depend on the variable with which sleep is being associated. Given the association between serotonin and both sleep and anxiety,[31,32] it is likely that genes involved in the serotonin pathways, and a host of others, are likely to play a role in any sleep-anxiety relationship. Complex phenotypes are likely to be influenced by multiple genes of small effect size, and therefore there is a need to further specify genes involved in sleep disturbances and associations with other traits. With the use of increasingly large-scale genome-wide association studies, it is likely that further candidates will soon emerge. Indeed, there have been three genome-wide association studies on subjective sleep phenotypes[33–35] that have highlighted candidates, some of which may be associated with internalizing difficulties.

Similarly, it is also necessary to specify environmental factors that account for the association between difficulties. Elements of the family and home environment are known to influence children's sleep and emotion. In their longitudinal study of infant sleep, Jansen and colleagues[25] found that certain parental behaviors (eg, the absence of set bedtimes, parental presence during sleep onset) preceded later emotional symptoms. It has been demonstrated that anxious parents are differentially involved in their children's bedtime routine.[36] Relative to those with nonanxious parents, the children of anxious parents were found to display disturbed sleep. Another study found that family disorganization and maternal depression each correlated moderately with sleep disturbance and anxiety symptoms in children aged 3 and 4 years and accounted for some of the association between the two difficulties.[37] Such findings emphasize the need to consider child sleep problems in the context of the family.[38]

Stress and trauma have also been implicated in altered biobehavioral functioning and have also been associated with psychopathology and sleep disorders.[39,40] Stressful life events or traumatic history could therefore be an additional bridge between sleep and psychopathology.

Genetic and environmental influences are commonly considered separately, but it is likely that they do not work independently but together to exert their effects. Indeed, interactions between genes and environmental factors are shown for difficulties including sleep quality[41] and various associated traits, including depression and behavioral difficulties.[42]

Pathways Through Which Genetic and Environmental Factors Work

In addition to understanding genetic and environmental influences on sleep disturbances and anxiety, further research needs to identify the pathways by which these influences have their effects. As described next, genetic and environmental factors are likely to impact on hormones and psychological processes known to be associated with sleep and emotional problems.

Hormonal Factors

In response to a perceived threat, the body releases stress hormones, including cortisol, which promote vigilance and prepare the individual for fight-or-flight behaviors.[43] These hormones are likely to have insomnogenic actions[44] and thus a state of arousal in the presleep period is likely to make sleep less likely. The hypothalamic-pituitary-adrenal axis, which controls reactivity to stress, is likely to be involved in the association between sleep and anxiety. In the study by Warren and colleagues,[36] the children of anxious parents were found to display elevated levels of cortisol and disturbed sleep. In addition, elevated presleep cortisol levels have been observed in children with anxiety disorders.[45]

Regulatory Systems

Dahl[46] outlines how sleep, arousal, and affect are overlapping regulatory systems, with dysregulation in one system impacting on the others: sleep disruption during critical developmental periods may increase the likelihood of later affective dysregulation and vice versa. For instance, disturbed sleep may disrupt processes occurring in the prefrontal cortex.[27] This area of the brain is known to be important in the executive functioning needed to control emotion and cognition.[47] Consequently, affected children might then be at risk of impaired emotional processing and potentially internalizing/externalizing disorders.

Indeed, studies have shown that a consequence of sleep disturbance is impaired affective regulation and coping skills. For example, otherwise healthy individuals demonstrate heightened negative affect following mild-to-moderate sleep deprivation.[48] Thus, anxious children may find their emotional difficulties heightened if they proceed to suffer from disrupted sleep.

Cognitive Processes

The cognitive model of insomnia[49] illustrates how particular dysfunctional cognitions concerning disturbed sleep may feed on themselves and exacerbate the problem. These cognitions, and the presence of a particular cognitive style that may predispose toward emotional difficulties, have primarily been researched in adults but are now receiving greater attention in young people. For example, in adults, presleep arousal has been investigated in adults in terms of somatic (ie, physiologic) and cognitive arousal, with both associated with disturbed sleep.[50] Of the two, cognitive arousal has been found to demonstrate the stronger association with sleep disruption, and this has been shown in community and clinical samples of youth.[2,11] Adults experiencing GAD have been found to report greater levels of cognitive activity and worry at bedtime, relative to nonanxious insomniacs and control subjects.[51] They also rated their presleep worries as less controllable and more interfering. Other research has considered the potential importance of specific cognitions and cognitive styles. For example, Alfano and colleagues[52] found that adolescents' sleep problems were correlated with "negative cognitive errors" (eg, internal attribution for negative outcomes, selective attendance to negative aspects of an event). Such beliefs are implicated in the development of anxiety and depression.[53] Similarly, the cognitive process of catastrophizing may also be of importance. This describes a particular cognitive style whereby individuals are prone to focus on the worst possible outcome of a situation, overestimate the chance that this will occur, and exaggerate the consequences of this occurrence.[54] Catastrophizing is known to be associated with anxiety[54] and has also been implicated in sleep disturbance.[55,56] Further exploration of the interplay between sleep, sleep-related cognitions, and anxiety is necessary.

SUMMARY

Anxiety and sleep difficulties are associated in youth. Indeed, the growing body of literature has shown that anxious children do not always sleep well and that in certain cases sleep disturbances in youth may serve as a red flag for the development of later anxiety. Whereas historically sleep disturbance has to some extent been dismissed as a symptom of other disorders, this view is becoming outdated. It is now acknowledged that sleep disturbances need to be considered in their own right. Indeed, in the *Diagnostic and Statistical Manual of Mental Disorders, 5th Edition*, the concept of "primary insomnia" and "insomnia related to another disorder" has been replaced by "insomnia disorder," which may or may not be comorbid with other disorders. Further research aimed at understanding the mechanisms between sleep disturbance and anxiety is of paramount importance and holds the promise of improving the quality of life for children and the families with whom they live.

REFERENCES

1. Leahy E, Gradisar M. Dismantling the bidirectional relationship between paediatric sleep and anxiety. Clin Psychol 2012;16(1):44–56.
2. Alfano CA, Pina AA, Zerr AA, et al. Pre-sleep arousal and sleep problems of anxiety-disordered youth. Child Psychiatry Hum Dev 2010;41(2):156–67.
3. Gregory AM, Caspi A, Moffitt TE, et al. Juvenile mental health histories of adults with anxiety disorders. Am J Psychiatry 2007;164(2):301–8.
4. Gregory AM, Sadeh A. Sleep, emotional and behavioral difficulties in children and adolescents. Sleep Med Rev 2012;16(2):129–36.
5. Gregory AM, Caspi A, Eley TC, et al. Prospective longitudinal associations between persistent sleep problems in childhood and anxiety and depression disorders in adulthood. J Abnorm Child Psychol 2005;33(2):157–63.
6. Gregory AM, O'Connor TG. Sleep problems in childhood: a longitudinal study of developmental change and association with behavioral problems. J Am Acad Child Adolesc Psychiatry 2002;41(8):964–71.
7. American Psychiatric Association. Diagnostic and statistical manual of mental disorders. 5th edition. Washington, DC: American Psychiatric Association; 2013.
8. American Academy of Sleep Medicine. International classification of sleep disorders: diagnostic and coding manual. 3rd edition. Westchester (IL): American Academy of Sleep Medicine; 2014.
9. Donker T, Petrie K, Proudfoot J, et al. Smartphones for smarter delivery of mental health programs: a systematic review. J Med Internet Res 2013;15(11):e247.
10. Touchette E, Chollet A, Galera C, et al. Prior sleep problems predict internalising problems later in life. J Affect Disord 2012;143(1–3):166–71.
11. Gregory AM, Willis TA, Wiggs L, et al. Presleep arousal and sleep disturbances in children. Sleep 2008;31(12):1745–7.
12. Gregory AM, Cousins JC, Forbes EE, et al. Sleep items in the child behavior checklist: a comparison with sleep diaries, actigraphy, and polysomnography. J Am Acad Child Adolesc Psychiatry 2011;50(5):499–507.
13. Owens JA, Spirito A, McGuinn M, et al. Sleep habits and sleep disturbance in elementary school-aged children. J Dev Behav Pediatr 2000;21(1):27–36.
14. Gregory AM, Rijsdijk FV, Dahl RE, et al. Associations between sleep problems, anxiety, and depression in twins at 8 years of age. Pediatrics 2006;118(3):1124–32.
15. Storch EA, Murphy TK, Lack CW, et al. Sleep-related problems in pediatric obsessive-compulsive disorder. J Anxiety Disord 2008;22(5):877–85.
16. Johnson EO, Chilcoat HD, Breslau N. Trouble sleeping and anxiety/depression in childhood. Psychiatry Res 2000;94(2):93–102.
17. Schredl M, Fricke-Oerkermann L, Mitschke A, et al. Longitudinal study of nightmares in children: stability and effect of emotional symptoms. Child Psychiatry Hum Dev 2009;40(3):439–49.
18. Mindell JA, Barrett KM. Nightmares and anxiety in elementary-aged children: is there a relationship. Child Care Health Dev 2002;28(4):317–22.
19. Alfano CA, Ginsburg GS, Kingery JN. Sleep-related problems among children and adolescents with anxiety disorders. J Am Acad Child Psychiatry 2007; 46(2):224–32.
20. Alfano CA, Beidel DC, Turner SM, et al. Preliminary evidence for sleep complaints among children referred for anxiety. Sleep Med 2006;7(6):467–73.
21. Rapoport J, Elkins R, Langer DH, et al. Childhood obsessive-compulsive disorder. Am J Psychiatry 1981;138(12):1545–54.
22. Forbes EE, Bertocci MA, Gregory AM, et al. Objective sleep in pediatric anxiety disorders and major depressive disorder. J Am Acad Child Adolesc Psychiatry 2008;47(2):148–55.
23. Alfano CA, Reynolds K, Scott N, et al. Polysomnographic sleep patterns of non-depressed, non-medicated children with generalized anxiety disorder. J Affect Disord 2013;147(1–3):379–84.
24. Shanahan L, Copeland WE, Angold A, et al. Sleep problems predict and are predicted by generalized anxiety/depression and oppositional defiant disorder. J Am Acad Child Adolesc Psychiatry 2014; 53(5):550–8.
25. Jansen P, Saridjan N, Hofman A, et al. Does disturbed sleeping precede symptoms of anxiety or depression in toddlers? the generation R study. Psychosom Med 2011;73(3):242–9.
26. Goldman-Mellor S, Gregory A, Caspi A, et al. Mental health antecedents of early midlife insomnia: evidence from a four-decade longitudinal study. Sleep 2014;37(11):1767–75.

27. Kelly RJ, El-Sheikh M. Reciprocal relations between children's sleep and their adjustment over time. Dev Psychol 2014;50(4):1137–47.

28. Plomin R, DeFries J, Knopik V, et al. Behavioral genetics. 6th edition. New York: Worth Publishers; 2014.

29. Van den Oord EJ, Boomsma DI, Verhulst FC. A study of genetic and environmental effects on the co-occurrence of problem behaviors in three-year-old twins. J Abnorm Psychol 2000;109(3):360–72.

30. Gehrman PR, Meltzer LJ, Moore M, et al. Heritability of insomnia symptoms in youth and their relationship to depression and anxiety. Sleep 2011; 34(12):1641–6.

31. Jouvet M. Biogenic amines and the states of sleep. Science 1969;163(3862):32–41.

32. Lesch KP, Bengel D, Heils A, et al. Association of anxiety-related traits with a polymorphism in the serotonin transporter gene regulatory region. Science 1996;274(5292):1527–31.

33. Allebrandt KV, Amin N, Muller-Myhsok B, et al. A K(ATP) channel gene effect on sleep duration: from genome-wide association studies to function in Drosophila. Mol Psychiatry 2013;18(1):122–32.

34. Byrne EM, Gehrman PR, Medland SE, et al. A genome-wide association study of sleep habits and insomnia. Am J Med Genet B Neuropsychiatr Genet 2013;162B(5):439–51.

35. Gottlieb DJ, O'Connor GT, Wilk JB. Genome-wide association of sleep and circadian phenotypes. BMC Med Genet 2007;8(Suppl 1):S9.

36. Warren SL, Gunnar MR, Kagan J, et al. Maternal panic disorder: infant temperament, neurophysiology, and parenting behaviors. J Am Acad Child Adolesc Psychiatry 2003;42(7):814–25.

37. Gregory AM, Eley TC, O'Connor TG, et al. Family influences on the association between sleep problems and anxiety in a large sample of pre-school aged twins. Pers Individ Dif 2005;39(8):1337–48.

38. Dahl RE, El-Sheikh M. Considering sleep in a family context: introduction to the special issue. J Fam Psychol 2007;21(1):1–3.

39. Charuvastra A, Cloitre M. Safe enough to sleep: sleep disruptions associated with trauma, posttraumatic stress, and anxiety in children and adolescents. Child Adolesc Psychiatr Clin N Am 2009; 18(4):877–91.

40. Sadeh A. Stress, trauma, and sleep in children. Child Adolesc Psychiatr Clin N Am 1996;5(3): 685–700.

41. Brummett BH, Krystal AD, Ashley-Koch A, et al. Sleep quality varies as a function of 5-HTTLPR genotype and stress. Psychosom Med 2007;69(7):621–4.

42. Moffitt TE, Caspi A, Rutter M. Strategy for investigating interactions between measured genes and measured environments. Arch Gen Psychiatry 2005;62(5):473–81.

43. Herman JP, Cullinan WE. Neurocircuitry of stress: central control of the hypothalamo-pituitary-adrenocortical axis. Trends Neurosci 1997;20(2): 78–84.

44. Richardson GS. Human physiological models of insomnia. Sleep Med 2007;8(Suppl 4):S9–14.

45. Forbes EE, Williamson DE, Ryan ND, et al. Perisleep-onset cortisol levels in children and adolescents with affective disorders. Biol Psychiatry 2006;59(1):24–30.

46. Dahl RE. The regulation of sleep and arousal: development and psychopathology. Dev Psychopathol 1996;8(1):3–27.

47. Muzur A, Pace-Schott EF, Hobson J. The prefrontal cortex in sleep. Trends Cogn Sci 2002;6(11):475–81.

48. Wolfson AR, Carskadon MA. Sleep schedules and daytime functioning in adolescents. Child Dev 1998;69(4):875–87.

49. Harvey AG. A cognitive model of insomnia. Behav Res Ther 2002;40(8):869–93.

50. Nicassio PM, Mendlowitz DR, Fussell JJ, et al. The phenomenology of the pre-sleep state: the development of the pre-sleep arousal scale. Behav Res Ther 1985;23(3):263–71.

51. Belanger L, Morin CM, Gendron L, et al. Presleep cognitive activity and thought control strategies in insomnia. J Cognit Psychother 2005;19(1):19–28.

52. Alfano CA, Zakem AH, Costa NM, et al. Sleep problems and their relation to cognitive factors, anxiety, and depressive symptoms in children and adolescents. Depress Anxiety 2009;26(6):503–12.

53. Weems CF, Costa NM, Watts SE, et al. Cognitive errors, anxiety sensitivity, and anxiety control beliefs: their unique and specific associations with childhood anxiety symptoms. Behav Modif 2007;31(2): 174–201.

54. Davey GC, Levy S. Catastrophic worrying: personal inadequacy and a perseverative iterative style as features of the catastrophizing process. J Abnorm Psychol 1998;107(4):576–86.

55. Barclay NL, Gregory AM. The presence of a perseverative iterative style in good vs. poor sleepers. J Behav Ther Exp Psychiatry 2010;41:18–23.

56. Willis TA, Yearall S, Gregory AM. Sleep quality and cognitive style in older adults. Cognit Ther Res 2011;35(1):1–10.

Sleep in Children and Adolescents with Obsessive-Compulsive Disorder

Katharine C. Reynolds, MA[a], Michael Gradisar, PhD[b],
Candice A. Alfano, PhD[a],*

KEYWORDS

- Obsessive-compulsive disorder • Anxiety disorder • Children • Adolescents • Sleep-onset latency
- Total sleep time • Presleep arousal • Bedtime resistance

KEY POINTS

- Sleep problems are not a core feature of obsessive-compulsive disorder (OCD), but emerging empirical data indicate some form of sleep disruption to be highly common.
- Available research in both adult and child patients is limited in several important ways, including the use of subjective reports (particularly in children), high rates of comorbid depression, and concurrent use of psychotropic medication.
- The presence of sleep disruption in OCD patients may compound severity and impairment of the disorder.
- More research is needed to fully understand the nature and consequences of sleep-wake disruption in children with OCD.

INTRODUCTION

OCD is a common and often disabling disorder with lifetime prevalence rates ranging from 2% to 3%.[1,2] It is the fourth most common psychiatric disorder in the population, diagnosed nearly as often as asthma.[3] OCD is characterized by the presence of recurrent intrusive thoughts or images (ie, obsessions) that seem excessive and/or irrational to an individual as well as behavioral rituals (ie, compulsions) directed at reducing associated anxiety. Collectively, these symptoms can cause marked distress, are unreasonably time consuming, and may significantly impair functioning in any or all aspects of life, including personal relationships, education, employment, finances, and health.[4,5]

Although OCD has been moved from the anxiety disorders section in the *Diagnostic and Statistical Manual for Mental Disorders* (Fourth Edition, Text Revision)[6] to the OCD and related disorders section in the *Diagnostic and Statistical Manual for Mental Disorders* (Fifth Edition) (**Box 1**), OCD patients nevertheless experience significant anxiety related to their disorder.[4,6]

Although not always able to understand or communicate their symptoms, children are just as likely as adults to suffer from OCD.[7,8] The disorder is sometimes seen in children as young as 4 and 5 years of age,[9] although most patients report an onset of symptoms during the school-age or early teenage years.[10] Like their adult counterparts, children with OCD commonly experience both

Funding Sources: None.
Conflict of Interest: None.
[a] Sleep and Anxiety Center of Houston, Department of Psychology, University of Houston, 126 Heyne Building, Houston, TX 77204, USA; [b] School of Psychology, Flinders University, GPO Box 2100, Adelaide, South Australia 5001, Australia
* Corresponding author.
E-mail address: caalfano@uh.edu

Box 1
Abbreviated *Diagnostic and Statistical Manual for Mental Disorders* (Fifth Edition) diagnostic criteria for obsessive-compulsive disorder

A. Presence of obsessions, compulsions, or both:

   Obsessions are defined by (1) and (2):

   1. Recurrent and persistent thoughts, urges, or images that are experienced, at some time during the disturbance, as intrusive and unwanted, and that in most individuals cause marked anxiety or distress

   2. An individual attempting to ignore or suppress such thoughts, urges, or images or to neutralize them with some other thought or action

   Compulsions are defined by (1) and (2):

   1. Repetitive behaviors that an individual feels driven to perform in response to an obsession or according to rules that must be applied rigidly

   2. The behaviors or mental acts are aimed at preventing or reducing anxiety or distress or preventing some dreaded event or situation; however, these behaviors or mental acts are not connected in a realistic way with what they are designed to neutralize or prevent, or are clearly excessive. Note: young children may not be able to articulate the aims of these behaviors or mental acts.

B. The obsessions or compulsions are time consuming (eg, >1 h/d) or cause clinically significant distress or impairment in social, occupational, or other important areas of functioning.

C. The obsessive-compulsive symptoms are not attributable to the physiologic effects of a substance (eg, a drug of abuse or a medication) or another medical condition.

D. The disturbance is not better explained by the symptoms of another mental disorder.

---

obsessions and compulsions. Children are more likely to present with compulsions/ritualized behaviors in the absence of specific obsessions.[11] The content of these behaviors varies considerably but frequently includes excessive hand washing or bathing; repeating certain numbers, words, or phrases; ordering items or doing something until it is "just right"; and checking behaviors.[11]

Despite that compulsions/rituals may consume up to several hours per day, children are sometimes able perform these behaviors in secret, hiding them from parents for extended periods.[11] As a result, parental reports of child obsessions and compulsions may underestimate both the severity and associated impairments of these symptoms.[12] In children, as in adults, interference across numerous areas of daily functioning may be present, such as in the ability to complete assigned tasks (ie, chores, homework, and schoolwork), in familial and social relationships (ie, getting along with parents, siblings, and friends), and in routines over the day and into the evening (ie, leaving for school, eating meals, and getting ready for bed). Functional impairments may also relate to problems with sleep, which are common[13,14] but poorly understood.

Sleep problems are not a core syndromal manifestation or prominent feature of OCD, yet empirical studies in children indicate some form of disruption to the sleep-wake cycle as highly common.[13,14] In the authors' child anxiety clinic, for example, children with OCD (or their parents) sometimes report a need to engage in time-consuming rituals before bed, which must be performed to their satisfaction prior to initiating sleep. Some children are unable to sleep in their own bed due to contamination fears, which results in a lack of a consistent sleep environment and routine. The sleep problems of children with OCD resemble those typically associated with other forms of childhood anxiety, including general nighttime fears, a need to cosleep, or lengthy sleep-onset latencies. The goal of this article is to provide a summary of available research examining the sleep patterns and problems associated with OCD. Because the existing body of literature focused on children specifically is limited, the discussion begins with a review of studies conducted among adult patients with OCD.

SLEEP IN ADULTS WITH OBSESSIVE-COMPULSIVE DISORDER

Although studies are limited compared with other psychiatric conditions, such as depression, examination of objective sleep patterns in OCD has produced inconsistent results. In an initial examination by Insel and colleagues,[15] 14 patients with OCD, 14 age-matched patients with depression, and 14 age- and gender-matched controls were compared on objective measures of sleep. Significantly reduced total sleep time (TST), more awakenings, reduced stage 4 sleep, and shortened latency to rapid eye movement (LREM) sleep were observed in OCD patients compared with controls. Although fewer significant differences emerged between the clinical groups, OCD patients exhibited significantly greater amounts of stages 1 and 3 sleep than depressed patients. A major limitation of this study, however, is that at least half of OCD patients had a secondary depressive disorder, and research based on subjective reports suggests that the sleep problems of OCD patients may actually derive from co-occurring depression.[16] For example, Bobdey and colleagues[16] examined 12 OCD patients without comorbid depression, 12 OCD patients with comorbid depression, 57 healthy control patients, and 13 patients with primary depression. Patients in both groups with a depressive diagnosis reported worse sleep than the 2 nondepressed groups, suggesting that depression rather than OCD adversely affects sleep.

Bobdey and colleagues[16] also examined sleep phase delay in their sample, with more mixed results. Specifically, among those subjects with bedtimes in the 90th percentile (ie, the latest bedtimes) were 2 patients with OCD without depression, 1 patient with OCD and depression, and 3 patients with depression only, pointing toward a higher incidence of sleep phase delay in all 3 clinical groups compared with controls. Similarly, Mukhopadhyay and colleagues[17] examined sleep circadian rhythms in OCD patients by sampling consecutive OCD-based inpatient admissions over a 10-year period. Of 187 eligible patients, 33 (17.6%) fulfilled criteria for delayed sleep phase syndrome (DSPS). All 33 patients had a significantly earlier age of OCD onset than OCD patients without DSPS. An additional 31% (n = 58) of patients reported sleep disturbances other than DSPS. Levels of comorbid depressive symptoms did not differ among OCD patients with and without any form of sleep disturbance. It is unclear how well results of this inpatient study generalize to nonhospitalized patients.

Hohagan and colleagues[18] examined 22 nonmedicated patients with OCD and 22 age-matched controls in terms of sleep, OCD severity (using the Yale-Brown Obsessive Compulsive Scale [Y-BOCS]),[19] and depression. Poorer sleep efficiency (SE) and an increased wake time during the sleep period were found in the OCD group. No

group differences were found for total rapid eye movement (REM) sleep, although the duration and density of the first REM period were nonsignificantly increased among OCD patients. Seven (32%) patients suffered from secondary depression and were, therefore, compared with nondepressed OCD patients on sleep variables. No differences were found. These findings are in line with those from previous studies (eg, including reduced SE and greater wake time) and suggest sleep disturbances to be related to a diagnosis of OCD.[15,20] Although Hohagan and colleagues[18] used a 7-day medication wash-out period,[21,22] other researchers have found increased REM density among OCD patients who have taken psychotropic medications previously compared with patients without a history of pharmacologic intervention.[23] As reported by Voderholzer and colleagues,[23] this difference could not be attributed to OCD severity or to comorbid depressive symptoms. The long-term effects of psychotropic medications on sleep are not yet understood.

The study by Voderholzer and colleagues[23] examined the sleep patterns of 62 nonmedicated patients with OCD and 62 matched healthy controls. The investigators noted that "many patients" in the OCD group had mild to moderate depressive symptoms secondary to OCD and only 29 of the patients had never been treated with psychotropic medication. Groups were compared on sleep continuity variables (ie, SE, sleep-onset latency, and number of awakenings) and sleep architecture (ie, LREM, duration of first REM period, and total REM density). Significant differences were seen on sleep variables between the groups, including shorter sleep duration, lower SE, and more time spent awake in the OCD group. Significant increases in REM density during the first REM period were also found among OCD subjects.

In a sample of 13 nonmedicated outpatients with OCD (who had each taken psychotropic medications previously) and a sample of matched controls, Robinson and colleagues[24] compared the sleep EEG of the 2 groups based on 2 nights of recording. No significant between-group differences were found for sleep measures. Within the OCD group, however, Y-BOCS scores were negatively correlated with TST, SE, and duration of sleep stages 1 and 2. Importantly, all patients in this sample were free of comorbid depressive diagnoses as well as significant depressive symptoms.

Kluge and colleagues[25] compared 10 inpatients with OCD (without comorbid depression) with 10 matched healthy controls using polysomnography (PSG). Sleep did not differ between the groups with the exception of reduced stage 4 sleep in

OCD patients, similar to results reported by Insel and colleagues.[15] In addition, LREM of less than 10 minutes was found among 3 individuals with OCD who had significantly more severe forms of the disorder compared with the other inpatients (as measured by the Y-BOCS). Although inpatients in this study did not have comorbid depression and were not taking medication at the time of participation, 3 subjects had previously been treated for a major depressive episode and all 10 inpatients had been on psychotropics at one time. The duration of drug-free intervals ranged from 9 days to several years.

SUMMARY OF ADULT-BASED STUDIES

For the most part, adult findings are largely limited by the potential influence of co-occurring depression, the unclear impact of psychotropic medications on sleep architecture, and the collection of objective sleep data under laboratory (ie, artificial) conditions. As a result, conclusions that can be drawn from these studies remain tenuous. These studies suggest similarities in the sleep of patients with OCD and patient with depressive symptoms, not necessarily accounted for by high rates of co-morbidity.[15,18,23,25] Similarities include poor SE, reduced slow wave sleep, increased wake after sleep onset (WASO), and a phase delay in the timing of sleep.

Despite similarities in presentation, sleep disturbances may hold different implications for these clinical groups. Whereas sleep deprivation (SD) produces (transient) improvements in mood in up to 70% of depressed patients,[26,27] the effects of SD on OCD symptoms seem more variable. In the only published study to use SD in a sample of 16 patients with OCD, findings included no change in OCD symptoms in 8 patients, improvement in 5 patients, and a worsening of symptoms in 3 patients.[28] Although the impact of co-occurring depression on SD outcomes is unclear, collectively, available data reveal a complex relationship between OCD symptoms and SD worthy of further investigation. Readers searching for more information about the relationship between OCD and sleep in adults are referred to a recent systematic review by Patterson and colleagues.[29]

SLEEP IN CHILDREN WITH OBSESSIVE-COMPULSIVE DISORDER

Sleep findings among adult OCD patients are equivocal; studies using objective sleep measures in children with OCD are relatively nonexistent. Most available studies have investigated the presence of sleep-related problems based on subjective child or parent reports. For example, Alfano and colleagues[13] found that 54% of children with primary OCD (ages 7 to 14 years) reported trouble sleeping and 64% reported difficulty waking in the morning. Among a larger sample, Storch and colleagues[14] found that, based on parent report, 90% of children and adolescents with OCD (ages 8 to 17 years) experienced some type of sleep-related problem including, most commonly, trouble sleeping and daytime tiredness. Sleep problems were more common in girls and younger children and were associated with more severe forms of OCD. In line with findings from Alfano and colleagues,[13] 44% of the sample experienced trouble sleeping, based on child reports. A limitation of the study by Storch and colleagues, however, includes that a majority of youth were taking psychotropic medications at the time of assessment.

Ivarsson and Larsson[30] conducted the largest study of sleep in youth with OCD to date, although also based on subjective reports. Three groups of Swedish children and adolescents were included: 185 inpatients with OCD (mean age = 12.9 y), 177 outpatients from a child and adolescent psychiatry clinic, and 317 controls from a normative school sample. Similar to methods used by Storch and colleagues,[14] sleep was assessed using items from the Child Behavior Checklist[31] based on parent report. As expected, significantly higher rates of sleep problems were found for the OCD and outpatient groups compared with controls. Approximately one-third of youth with OCD and one-fifth of the outpatient group were reported to have a sleep-related problem, although this difference was nonsignificant. Ivarsson and Larsson's[30] study had a large sample size and included a normal comparison group, which extends this research literature. Investigations of sleep using objective measures in children with OCD remain, however, largely unavailable.

In the only published study to use laboratory-based PSG in youth, Rapoport and colleagues[32] compared the sleep of 9 adolescents with OCD (ages 13–17 years) to a group of matched healthy controls. Three subjects with OCD met diagnostic criteria for major depressive disorder at the time of assessment, all patients had a history of depression, and 5 of the 9 patients had been treated with psychotropic medication in the past. Findings included significantly reduced SE and increased SOL within the OCD group; these adolescents required twice as long as controls to initiate sleep onset. Additionally, OCD patients had an average TST of 363 minutes (standard deviation = 58) compared with 421 minutes (standard deviation = 40) among controls.

A pilot study by Alfano and Kim[33] compared the sleep of a small group of nonmedicated, nondepressed children with OCD (n = 6) to a group of matched healthy control children, all aged 7 to 11 years. All children wore wrist actigraphs at home for 7 consecutive days. Actigraphy results indicated significantly reduced TST and increased WASO among youth with OCD. More specifically, the OCD group averaged 389 (standard deviation = 32) minutes of TST per night across the 1-week period compared with an average of 480 (standard deviation = 21.5) minutes for controls. Although the 2 groups did not differ in terms of total number of nighttime awakenings, duration of arousals was twice as long in the clinical group. Comparable with adult-based findings reported by Robinson and colleagues,[24] a significant negative association was found between TST and severity of compulsions as measured by the Children's Y-BOCS.[34] These data suggest that sleep problems may emerge early in the development of OCD and are not attributable to the effects of medication or secondary depression. Based on the study's small sample size, however, replication of these findings is necessary.

Finally, in an attempt to understand potential processes involved in the interplay between OCD and sleep, Alfano and colleagues[13] measured both cognitive and somatic presleep arousal in 52 anxious children and adolescents (7–14 y), including 13 patients with OCD. Although cognitive presleep arousal was found significantly higher than somatic arousal in the anxious sample as a whole, surprisingly both forms of presleep arousal were not significantly related to either bedtime resistance or sleep latency. Instead, presleep cognitive arousal showed a significantly moderate relationship with TST, such that the higher the arousal the less TST was reported. Previous objective evidence has shown higher perisleep-onset cortisol levels in anxious children compared with healthy controls,[35] thus supporting Alfano and colleagues'[13] subjective reports of arousal prior to sleep. As much as the link between presleep arousal and lengthened sleep latency sounds plausible, however, evidence is needed in pediatric samples to support this link.

SUMMARY ON PEDIATRIC FINDINGS

Sleep plays a critical role in early development.[36] For youth with OCD, sleep problems during this period may compound the severity and burden of their illness. Unfortunately, the majority of available sleep research has been conducted in adult OCD patients, rendering unclear implications for children based on salient development differences in both OCD and sleep patterns during this period. Adult-based studies are also limited by high rates of comorbidity. Yet, because adult patients are more likely to meet criteria for a comorbid depressive disorder,[37] childhood may afford an important window for better understanding the unique linkages between OCD psychopathology and sleep.

Of the few studies that have focused on children with OCD, subjectively reported sleep problems are prevalent.[13,14] Two published studies have used objective sleep methods and provide evidence of reduced TST in youth despite the use of different measurement techniques and age ranges.[32,33] Other objective sleep findings include reduced SE, increased SOL, and increased WASO. Research aimed at replicating these findings is a necessary next step, including investigations that compare subjective sleep reports with objective outcomes. The potential role of comorbidity and the effects of psychotropic medications on sleep also require empirical attention.

From a clinical standpoint, evidence for a link between sleep problems and a more severe form of OCD in children[14,33] may have important implications for intervention. Despite descriptive data that provide insight into the ways in which obsessions and compulsions each relate to difficulties during the presleep and sleep periods, more and better data are needed. Neurobiological mechanisms underlying this association also remain speculative at present. As a possible foci for future research in this area, Alfano and Kim[33] have hypothesized that because insufficient sleep, particularly during childhood, most profoundly affects executive functions of the prefrontal cortex,[38] including behavioral and emotional inhibition, obsessions and compulsions may become more difficult to resist (ie, inhibit) when sleep is inadequate. Experimental designs that seek to directly test this possibility may provide guidance for researchers and clinicians alike. Fig. 1 presents a model synthesizing evidenced-based associations and hypothesizes links between factors that may help explain a vicious cycle occurring during comorbid OCD and sleep disturbance in children. More research is needed to confirm these associations.

TREATMENT OF SLEEP PROBLEMS COMORBID WITH PEDIATRIC OBSESSIVE-COMPULSIVE DISORDER

The gold-standard nonpharmacologic treatment of OCD in adults and children is cognitive behavior therapy (CBT).[39,40] CBT has also been found to augment treatment outcomes for pediatric OCD where medical management (ie, selective serotonin reuptake inhibitors) is used.[41] Unfortunately,

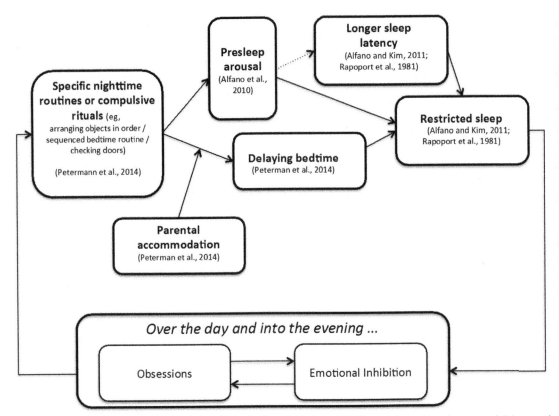

Fig. 1. A maintenance model for the comorbid relationship between OCD and sleep disturbance in children and adolescents.

data on whether CBT improves comorbid sleep problems in children and adolescents are lacking. There is recent recognition of a need for "empirical evaluation of underlying mechanisms and shared treatment effects for anxiety and sleep in youth."[42] In adults, the empirical evidence for shared treatment effects between sleep and OCD is small but nevertheless emerging. Using a nonpharmacologic sleep intervention, Abe and colleagues[43] treated the acute insomnia of a 25-year-old man with OCD using a combination of sleep hygiene (ie, moderating alcohol and caffeine consumption and regularizing habits across weekdays and weekends) and sleep perception training (ie, comparing actigraphic records of sleep with subjective reports). Abe and colleagues[43] report that the man's "anxiety and fear of insomnia diminished," although standardized changes in these outcomes do not seem to have been formally assessed.

In children, the evidence for shared treatment effects is slightly better than that in adult samples. Compared with a waitlist control group, Paine and Gradisar[44] found that OCD symptoms significantly decreased in school-aged children (7–12 y) diagnosed with behavioral insomnia in response to a

6-session CBT. These reductions in OCD occurred despite the focus of therapy on separation anxiety issues experienced by the sample, many of whom often needed parental presence to fall asleep. CBT consisted of treatment components seen in CBT for anxiety disorders (ie, cognitive restructuring, exposure therapy, and relaxation training). It also incorporated, however, treatment components extrapolated from CBT for adult insomnia (eg, sleep hygiene and bedtime fading [restriction therapy]). This randomized controlled trial provides some evidence of shared treatment reductions in OCD and sleep in children. Due to the multicomponent nature of the CBT used, however, the unique effect of sleep or anxiety treatment techniques on OCD is not known nor are the underlying mechanisms.[42]

Storch and colleagues[14] examined the effect of family-based CBT (ie, at least 1 parent attended all the sessions with the patient) for pediatric OCD on sleep-related problems. A total of 41 youth received weekly treatment over 14 weeks. Each session was 90 minutes in length, and core treatment components included psychoeducation, cognitive training, and exposure with response prevention.[14] Although sleep was not addressed directly, children demonstrated a significant

> **Box 2**
> **Interventions for comorbid pediatric obsessive-compulsive disorder and sleep problems**
>
> - Sleep hygiene—caffeine consumption can be reduced (eg, perform a caffeine diary that includes chocolate, soda, and tea); arousing pre-bedtime activities (eg, surfing the Internet) are replaced by relaxing techniques (eg, reading). Bedtimes and wake-up bedtimes are regularized across the school week and weekend, allowing for a predictable build-up of sleep pressure.
> - Bedtime fading—for children with a long sleep latency, bedtime may be gradually delayed until sleep latency is reduced to an acceptable level. Wake-up time needs to be consistent during the bedtime fading technique.
> - Stimulus control—if sleep latency is extended over 15–20 min, the child can sit up and read in bed or in a chair next to the bed for 10–15 min and then reattempt sleep. Repeat this process. This technique is best begun on a weekend night (eg, Friday).
> - Sleep restriction—in extreme circumstances, sleep restriction may be indicated. The child is recommended to spend time in bed 30 min less than the estimated TST. This should reduce wakefulness in bed, and sleepiness in the evening may reduce presleep arousal. This technique is best trialed during school holidays.

reduction in the total number of sleep-related problems post-treatment. Additionally, specific (parent-reported) problems of nightmares, sleeping less than most kids, being overtired, sleeping more than most kids, trouble sleeping, and sleeping next to someone else in the family all showed significant decreases from pre-to post-treatment. Thus, family-based CBT may be effective in reducing not only OCD symptoms[45] but also sleep-related problems in this population of youth.[14]

Across the aforementioned studies, sleep hygiene seems the most common treatment component applied.[43,45] Sleep hygiene has been suggested as a potential countermeasure to the theorized poor sleep hygiene that may be present in youth experiencing sleep problems comorbid with anxiety disorders.[42] There is a consensus by the American Academy of Sleep Medicine that sleep hygiene is not a recommended sole treatment of adults experiencing insomnia, yet it is simultaneously acknowledged that sleep hygiene is often an adjunct to other evidence-based techniques (eg, CBT for insomnia).[46] The authors extend the suggestion to use sleep hygiene in the treatment of childhood OCD and sleep problems to include additional behavioral sleep medicine treatment components. **Box 2** outlines each of these and how they align with the maintaining factors in **Fig. 1**.

Recent evidence suggests impairments in executive function are related to pediatric OCD,[42,47] and specifically that children low in emotional control receive the poorest treatment outcomes.[47] Therefore, any implementation of a sleep intervention for pediatric OCD comorbid with sleep problems should be mindful of factors moderating treatment outcome.

SUMMARY

Subjective and objective measurement of sleep in children and adolescents experiencing OCD demonstrates a longer time taken to fall asleep (sleep-onset latency) and restricted total sleep duration that may also include frequent night awakenings. Presleep arousal may be implicated in such sleep disturbances, yet more research is needed to confirm this link. Although models have been presented to understand the relationship between sleep problems and anxiety in school-aged children,[42] the authors present a framework for understanding the maintenance of pediatric OCD and sleep disturbance. The published literature is lacking directions for clinicians to treat both sleep problems and OCD using behavioral sleep medicine techniques. The authors present suggestions in this article (see **Box 2**) for clinicians to trial. These techniques also require, however, scientific validation, so that an evidence base may be established to help children and their families deal with the daily and nightly interference of OCD on their lives.

REFERENCES

1. Karno M, Golding JM, Sorenson SB, et al. The epidemiology of obsessive-compulsive disorder in five US communities. Arch Gen Psychiatry 1988; 45:1094–9.
2. Ruscio AM, Stein DJ, Chiu WT, et al. The epidemiology of obsessive-compulsive disorder in the National Comorbidity Survey Replication. Mol Psychiatry 2010;15:53–63.
3. Hollander E, Stein D. Obsessive–compulsive disorders: etiology, diagnosis, treatment. New York: Marcel Decker; 1997.

4. American Psychiatric Association. Diagnostic and statistic manual of mental disorders (DSM-5). Washington, DC: American Psychiatric Association; 2013.

5. Koran LM, Thienemann ML, Davenport R. Quality of life for patients with obsessive-compulsive disorder. Am J Psychiatry 1996;153:783–8.

6. American Psychiatric Association. Diagnostic and statistical manual of mental disorders: DSM-IV-TR. 4th edition. Washington, DC: American Psychiatric Association; 2000.

7. Flament M, Whitaker A, Rapoport J, et al. Obsessive compulsive disorder in adolescents: an epidemiological study. J Am Acad Child Adolesc Psychiatry 1988;27:764–71.

8. Geller D, Biederman J, Jones J, et al. Is juvenile obsessive-compulsive disorder a developmental subtype of the disorder? A review of the pediatric literature. J Am Acad Child Adolesc Psychiatry 1998;37:420–7.

9. Beidel D, Alfano C. Child anxiety disorders: a guide to research and treatment. 2nd edition. New York: Routledge; 2011.

10. Rasmussen SA, Eisen JL. The epidemiology and differential diagnosis of obsessive compulsive disorder. J Clin Psychiatry 1992;53(Suppl):4–10.

11. Swedo SE, Rapoport JL, Leonard H, et al. Obsessive-compulsive disorder in children and adolescents. Clinical phenomenology of 70 consecutive cases. Arch Gen Psychiatry 1989;46:335–41.

12. Rapoport JL, Inoff-Germain G, Weissman MM, et al. Childhood obsessive-compulsive disorder in the NIMH MECA study: parent versus child identification of cases. Methods for the epidemiology of child and adolescent mental disorders. J Anxiety Disord 2000; 14:535–48.

13. Alfano CA, Pina AA, Zerr AA, et al. Pre-sleep arousal and sleep problems of anxiety-disordered youth. Child Psychiatry Hum Dev 2010;41:156–67.

14. Storch EA, Murphy TK, Lack CW, et al. Sleep-related problems in pediatric obsessive-compulsive disorder. J Anxiety Disord 2008;22:877–85.

15. Insel TR, Gillin JC, Moore A, et al. The sleep of patients with obsessive-compulsive disorder. Arch Gen Psychiatry 1982;39:1372–7.

16. Bobdey M, Fineberg N, Gale TM, et al. Reported sleep patterns in obsessive compulsive disorder (OCD). Int J Psychiatry Clin Pract 2002;6:15–21.

17. Mukhopadhyay S, Fineberg NA, Drummond LM, et al. Delayed sleep phase in severe obsessive-compulsive disorder: a systematic case-report survey. CNS Spectr 2008;13:406–13.

18. Hohagen F, Lis S, Krieger S, et al. Sleep EEG of patients with obsessive-compulsive disorder. Eur Arch Psychiatry Clin Neurosci 1994;243:273–8.

19. Goodman WK, Price LH, Rasmussen SA, et al. The Yale-Brown obsessive compulsive scale. I. Development, use, and reliability. Arch Gen Psychiatry 1989;46:1006–11.

20. Walsleben J, Robinson D, Lemus C, et al. Polysomnographic aspects of obsessive-compulsive disorders. Sleep Res 1990;19:177.

21. Berger M, Lund R, Bronisch T, et al. REM latency in neurotic and endogenous depression and the cholinergic REM induction test. Psychiatry Res 1983;10:113–23.

22. Lauer CJ, Pollmächer T. On the issue of drug washout prior to polysomnographic studies in depressed patients. Neuropsychopharmacology 1992;6:11–6.

23. Voderholzer U, Riemann D, Huwig-Poppe C, et al. Sleep in obsessive compulsive disorder: polysomnographic studies under baseline conditions and after experimentally induced serotonin deficiency. Eur Arch Psychiatry Clin Neurosci 2007;257:173–82.

24. Robinson D, Walsleben J, Pollack S, et al. Nocturnal polysomnography in obsessive-compulsive disorder. Psychiatry Res 1998;80:257–63.

25. Kluge M, Schüssler P, Dresler M, et al. Sleep onset REM periods in obsessive compulsive disorder. Psychiatry Res 2007;152:29–35.

26. Wirz-Justice A, Van den Hoofdakker RH. Sleep deprivation in depression: what do we know, where do we go? Biol Psychiatry 1999;46:445–53.

27. Wu JC, Bunney WE. The biological basis of an antidepressant response to sleep deprivation and relapse: review and hypothesis. Am J Psychiatry 1990;147:14–21.

28. Joffe RT, Swinson RP. Total sleep deprivation in patients with obsessive-compulsive disorder. Acta Psychiatr Scand 1988;77:483–7.

29. Paterson JL, Reynolds AC, Ferguson SA, et al. Sleep and obsessive-compulsive disorder (OCD). Sleep Med Rev 2013;17:465–74.

30. Ivarsson T, Larsson B. Sleep problems as reported by parents in Swedish children and adolescents with obsessive-compulsive disorder (OCD), child psychiatric outpatients and school children. Nord J Psychiatry 2009;63:480–4.

31. Achenbach TM. Ten-year comparisons of problems and competencies for national samples of youth: self, patent and teacher reports. J Emot Behav Disord 2002;10:194–203.

32. Rapoport J, Elkins R, Langer DH, et al. Childhood obsessive-compulsive disorder. Am J Psychiatry 1981;138:1545–54.

33. Alfano CA, Kim KL. Objective sleep patterns and severity of symptoms in pediatric obsessive compulsive disorder: a pilot investigation. J Anxiety Disord 2011;25:835–9.

34. Scahill L, Riddle MA, McSwiggin-Hardin M, et al. Children's Yale-Brown obsessive compulsive scale: reliability and validity. J Am Acad Child Adolesc Psychiatry 1997;36:844–52.

35. Forbes EE, Williamson DE, Ryan ND, et al. Peri-sleep-onset cortisol levels in children and adolescents with affective disorders. Biol Psychiatry 2006;59:24–30.

36. Dahl RE. The regulation of sleep and arousal: development and psychopathology. Development and Psychopathology 1996;8:3–27.

37. Mancebo MC, Garcia AM, Pinto A, et al. Juvenile-onset OCD: clinical features in children, adolescents and adults. Acta Psychiatr Scand 2008;118:149–59.

38. Muzur A, Pace-Schott EF, Hobson JA. The prefrontal cortex in sleep. Trends Cogn Sci 2002;6:475–81.

39. Peris TS, Piacentini J. Optimizing treatment for complex cases of childhood obsessive compulsive disorder: a preliminary trial. J Clin Child Adolesc Psychol 2013;42:1–8.

40. Hofmann SG, Smits JA. Cognitive-behavioral therapy for adult anxiety disorders: a meta-analysis of randomized placebo-controlled trials. J Clin Psychiatry 2008;69:621–32.

41. Franklin ME, Sapyta J, Freeman JB, et al. Cognitive behavior therapy augmentation of pharmacotherapy in pediatric obsessive-compulsive disorder: the Pediatric OCD Treatment Study II (POTS II) randomized controlled trial. JAMA 2011;306:1224–32.

42. Peterman JS, Carper MM, Kendall PC. Anxiety disorders and comorbid sleep problems in school-aged youth: review and future research directions. Child Psychiatry Hum Dev 2014. [Epub ahead of print].

43. Abe Y, Nishimura G, Endo T. Early sleep psychiatric intervention for acute insomnia: implications from a case of obsessive-compulsive disorder. J Clin Sleep Med 2012;8:191–3.

44. Paine S, Gradisar M. A randomised controlled trial of cognitive-behaviour therapy for behavioural insomnia of childhood in school-aged children. Behav Res Ther 2011;49:379–88.

45. Storch EA, Geffken GR, Merlo LJ, et al. Family-based cognitive-behavioral therapy for pediatric obsessive-compulsive disorder: comparison of intensive and weekly approaches. J Am Acad Child Adolesc Psychiatry 2007;46:469–78.

46. Morgenthaler T, Kramer M, Alessi C, et al. Practice parameters for the psychological and behavioral treatment of insomnia: an update. an American academy of sleep medicine report. Sleep 2006;29:1415–9.

47. McNamara J, Reid A, Balkhi A, et al. Self-regulation and other executive functions relationship to pediatric OCD severity and treatment outcome. J Psychopathol Behav Assess 2014;36:1–11.

Attention Deficit/ Hyperactivity Disorder and Sleep in Children

John H. Herman, PhD

KEYWORDS

- Attention deficit/hyperactivity disorder • Obstructive sleep apnea
- Periodic limb movement disorder • Sleep apnea

KEY POINTS

- ADHD is well known to be associated with sleep problems; problems with attention and hyperactivity are known manifestations of sleepiness in children.
- ADHD may be associated with objectively recorded sleep disruption.
- ADHD may be associated with excessive daytime sleepiness.
- ADHD is frequently associated with a comorbid psychiatric diagnosis in which case the comorbid condition is associated with disrupted sleep.
- Obstructive sleep apnea, snoring, and periodic limb movement disorder, are associated with ADHD.
- Stimulant medication in children with ADHD may disrupt sleep.
- Melatonin, and not zolpidem, is effective in treating sleeping problems in children with ADHD.
- ADHD often appears comorbidly with anxiety, depression, or bipolar disorder.
- Children with ADHD frequently have mild sleep apnea. Treating the sleep apnea with adenotonsillectomy alleviates the symptoms of ADHD more than stimulants without the undesirable side effects.

INTRODUCTION

Attention deficit/hyperactivity disorder (ADHD) is a psychiatric diagnosis that describes symptoms including hyperactivity, inattentiveness, and impulsivity of sufficient magnitude to impair normal functioning in children and adults. It is a common syndrome in children and in some cases persists in adults. The Diagnostic and Statistical Manual of Mental Disorders-IV, describes how 6 of 9 symptoms must be present to describe either the inattentive type or the hyperactive type. If an individual meets criteria for both, he or she is diagnosed with the combined type.

The manual also describes how most of the symptoms of ADHD are common in normal children; therefore, symptoms must persist for at least 6 months and must be present in more than one setting. For example, a child who meets ADHD criteria at home but not at school or vice versa would not meet criteria for ADHD. The symptoms must emerge before age 7. The symptoms cannot be explained by another mental disorder, such as depression, anxiety, or bipolar disorder.

In children especially, hyperactivity and difficulties with attention are common manifestations of insufficient sleep. A recent study found that 1 hour of sleep restriction for 6 nights in children with subclinical ADHD pushed two-thirds into the clinically impaired range on a test of daytime performance.[1]

University of Texas Southwestern Medical Center at Dallas, 5323 Harry Hines Boulevard, Dallas, TX 75390, USA
E-mail address: remsleep@sbcglobal.net

Sleep Med Clin 10 (2015) 143–149
http://dx.doi.org/10.1016/j.jsmc.2015.02.003
1556-407X/15/$ – see front matter © 2015 Elsevier Inc. All rights reserved.

The 2004 National Sleep Foundation's *Sleep in America* poll of children found that 1 in 4 parents reported that their child was not getting enough sleep and two-thirds reported that their child had one or more sleep problems a few nights a week.[2] These findings suggest that many vulnerable children may inadvertently be pressured into hyperactivity by chronic insufficient sleep. Such a sleep-deprived, tired, hyperactive or inattentive child is then prescribed a stimulant to ameliorate his or her symptoms, obviously not a desired treatment.

This article discusses how children with insufficient sleep, or with sleep disorders such as restless legs syndrome/periodic limb movement disorder (PLMD), or obstructive sleep apnea are more likely to manifest symptoms of ADHD. Children with insufficient sleep may exhibit hyperactivity and impulsivity, leading to the diagnosis of ADHD. This article also discusses the findings and controversies linking sleep difficulties to ADHD. It reviews current pharmacologic and nonpharmacologic treatments for ADHD.

A vast array of nonmedical literature addresses the diagnosis and treatment of ADHD from psychiatric, psychoanalytic, behavioral, and dietary perspectives. There are many publications in psychiatric, psychological, and nutritional journals and many textbooks addressing ADHD and its treatment that are outside of the medical literature These journal articles and textbooks inform health care professionals in school and workplace settings. Sleep issues appear principally in the medical literature. Psychological/behavioral issues appear mainly in the nonmedical literature. Entering the search terms "ADHD" and "sleep" in PubMed pulls up 743 journal articles. Entering the search term "ADHD" in the "books" category of Amazon.com pulls up more than 5000 publications. In scanning the first 100 publications at Amazon.com, there was no obvious overlap with its search results and those of PubMed. This article focuses exclusively on ADHD and sleep, a topic given scant notice in the nonmedical literature.

IS THE SLEEP OF CHILDREN WITH ATTENTION DEFICIT/HYPERACTIVITY DISORDER DISTURBED?

This question is surprisingly difficult to answer definitively. A recent meta-analysis concluded that parents of children with ADHD perceive them to have more bedtime resistance, more difficulty falling asleep, more nighttime awakenings, greater difficulty waking up in the morning, and more daytime sleepiness. Parents of ADHD children also report that they snore more than controls. The same analysis also reviewed results of polysomnography and actigraphy for more objective measures. This analysis found increased sleep-onset latency on actigraphy, more stage shifts per hour, lower sleep efficiency on polysomnography, and shorter total sleep time.[3] However, another meta-analysis of polysomnographic studies found no differences between ADHD children and controls with the exception that children with ADHD had more periodic leg movements (PLMs) than controls.[4]

The journal articles in PubMed were reviewed, comparing the sleep of normal controls with sleep of children of the same age with ADHD. No single objective abnormality characterizes the sleep of children with ADHD compared with controls. The subjective (parent reported) variable of increased bedtime resistance consistently differentiates children with ADHD from controls.[5] But actigraphy[6,7] and polysomnographic studies[8] do not corroborate longer latencies to sleep onset or shorter total sleep times or increased arousals in children with ADHD.

Studies of children with ADHD have been performed by questionnaire, by parents filling out logs, by actigraphy, and by polysomnography (PSG). Many use more than one of the above measurement techniques. Several studies find the sleep of children to be the same as control children by PSG or by actigraphy. Several studies find parental questionnaires to indicate sleep-onset problems and sleep maintenance problems in children with ADHD,[9] but PSG studies fail to verify this. Many PSG and actigraphy studies find a difference between children with ADHD and normal controls, but the differences between children with ADHD and normal controls are not consistent from one publication to the next. For example, several studies have found shorter sleep or greater wake after sleep onset in children with ADHD. Other studies report longer sleep in children with ADHD then controls. There are more publications that describe some form of sleep disorder, albeit different in each publication, than there are publications that describe no sleep abnormalities.

About the same number of publications reports no differences comparing children with ADHD with controls, and one reports longer total sleep time in children with ADHD as measured by actigraphy. Others report differences in rapid eye movement (REM) latency or total REM sleep time only.

Even if the sleep of children with ADHD is not different from that of normal controls, it does not rule out the possibility that both groups are sleep deprived to some extent but that children with ADHD are more vulnerable to sleep deprivation.

Given the findings from the National Sleep Foundation's 1994 poll of children's sleep, and their report of insufficient sleep in a sizable proportion of children, this explanation is distinctly plausible.

Another possible explanation is the high proportion of children with ADHD that have comorbid sleep disorders including OSA, PLMD/restless legs syndrome, and insomnia. It makes sense that children with sleep disorders are more likely to meet criteria for ADHD. If all children with any sleep disorders were removed from analysis, it is possible that the differences between ADHD children would become insignificantly small.

SLEEP DISORDERS AND ATTENTION DEFICIT/ HYPERACTIVITY DISORDER

The previous section postulated that the controversy in the relationship between ADHD and sleep quality might be resolved by eliminating all children with comorbid sleep disorders before examining sleep and ADHD. This section examines the relationship between sleep disorders and ADHD. The nature and strength of this relationship is also controversial.

For example, some studies report a relationship between snoring in children and ADHD.[10–12] Other studies do not find a relationship between snoring and OSA in children with ADHD.[13] When it comes to PLMD/restless legs syndrome, most but not all studies report a link to ADHD.[14,15] One study found that only PLMs with arousals were associated with ADHD, whereas PLMs without arousals were not.[14] But in the first section of this article, it was shown that some studies did not find increased arousals in ADHD,[8] which would appear to argue against the increased arousal-ADHD hypothesized link.

Some studies found sleep onset or sleep maintenance insomnia, increased awakenings, and decreased REM sleep in children with ADHD.[5] Other studies found one or more of these abnormalities, but few findings overlapped with those of other studies. Still other studies of sleep in ADHD reported subjective reports from parents of disrupted sleep that were not confirmed either by actigraphy in some cases and polysomnography.[6–8]

THE QUESTION OF EXCESSIVE DAYTIME SLEEPINESS AND ATTENTION DEFICIT/ HYPERACTIVITY DISORDER

The symptoms of hyperactivity or inattention are frequently linked to sleep deprivation in children. The National Sleep Foundation states that ADHD is linked to excessive daytime sleepiness (EDS).[16] Some studies report that children with

ADHD fall asleep on the standard test for EDS, the multiple sleep latency test (MSLT), more quickly than do controls.[17] Other studies of EDS using the MSLT in children find no differences in sleep latency.[18] One study using polysomnography to study nocturnal sleep and parent questionnaires to assess daytime sleepiness in children with ADHD compared with controls found no difference in EDS between groups.[8]

One study reports EDS only in the inattentive subtype of ADHD and not in the hyperactive or combined types.[19] One polysomnographic study suggests that ADHD is one of several neurocognitive sequelae of EDS.[20] This study compared unmedicated children with ADHD with those taking immediate-release methylphenidate and found the unmedicated children to have significant EDS and learning and behavioral issues.

Another study approached the question of EDS slightly differently. This study examined objective neurocognitive measures and parent-reported learning, attention/hyperactivity, and conduct problems in children with and without parent-reported EDS. In a large sample, about 15% of children were reported to have EDS. Structural equation modeling, a statistical technique to estimate causal relations, was used to examine whether processing speed and working memory performance would help explain the relationship between EDS and learning, attention/hyperactivity, and conduct problems. Logistic regression models, used to explain children's neurocognitive problems based on EDS, suggest that parent-reported learning, attention/hyperactivity, and conduct problems as well as objective measurement of processing speed and working memory are significantly associated with EDS, even when controlling for Apnea–Hypopnea Index (AHI) and objective markers of sleep.[20]

It is difficult to reconcile the mixed experimental findings with the frequently observed relationship between restricted sleep and inattentiveness/hyperactivity. In fact, one study restricted prepubertal children's sleep for 1 hour for 6 consecutive nights and tested them for ADHD severity and vigilance performance before and after restriction. This study had both an ADHD group and a normal control group. The authors reported that both normal controls and ADHD children performed more poorly after sleep restriction on vigilance tests, and the ADHD group's scores on a test of ADHD severity deteriorated from subclinical levels to the clinical range of inattention.[1] Another study compared normal children in 3 conditions: optimized sleep, normal sleep, and restricted sleep. The study found significant declines comparing the 3 conditions for academic problems, sleepiness, and attention.[21] Another study found sleep restriction in normal children was associated with shorter daytime sleep latency on the MSLT, increased subjective sleepiness, and increased sleepy and inattentive behavior but was not associated with increased hyperactivity, impulsive behavior, or impaired performance on tests of sustained attention.[22]

It seems as if sleep restriction in normal children or children with ADHD more consistently leads to daytime sleepiness then is demonstrated in studies of sleepiness in children with ADHD compared with normal controls. Perhaps the common perception of sleep restriction being associated with ADHD symptoms is related to parents observing children who have undergone one or more nights of sleep restriction and parents of children with ADHD observing them deteriorate with sleep restriction. Finally, it seems that EDS in children, with or without ADHD, leads to learning problems, behavioral issues, inattention, and hyperactivity.

ATTENTION DEFICIT/HYPERACTIVITY DISORDER COMORBID WITH OTHER PSYCHIATRIC DIAGNOSES

ADHD is frequently comorbid with other psychiatric disorders such as autism, mental retardation, anxiety, depression, and oppositional defiant disorder. In publications discussing comorbidity of ADHD with other psychiatric disorders, frequently the sleep of children with ADHD alone does not differ from that of controls, but those with comorbid psychiatric conditions frequently have more disordered sleep. One study examined sleep in subtypes of ADHD children with and without other psychiatric comorbidities. This study found that sleep in the inattentive type of ADHD did not differ from control children but that the sleep of children with both inattention and hyperactivity differed from controls as did the sleep of children with comorbid anxiety or depression. This study found the sleep of children with both ADHD and comorbid oppositional defiant disorder did not differ from controls.[23] Another study found that comorbid anxiety but not depression in children with ADHD increased sleep disorders but that both anxiety and depression increased sleep latency in children with ADHD.[24]

PHARMACOLOGIC TREATMENT OF ATTENTION DEFICIT/HYPERACTIVITY DISORDER

ADHD is most commonly treated with stimulant medication. Methylphenidate is used most commonly, but other stimulants, including amphetamine and dexamphetamine, are also used to treat ADHD. The nonstimulant, atomoxetine, is also used to treat ADHD. Methylphenidate is associated with sleep difficulty,[25] insomnia,[26] less total sleep time and less non-REM sleep,[27] and sleep disorders.[28] Each of the aforementioned references ascribes a sleep problem related to use of methylphenidate in children with ADHD, but no 2 report the same sleep problem. Some of the descriptors are vague, such as sleep difficulty or sleep disorder. Others could overlap. Not one replicates another.

Then there is the question of dose and timing of administration. One study reports increased insomnia with increased dose of methylphenidate,[26] another reports that the duration of wearing a methylphenidate transdermal patch had no effect on sleep latency or total sleep time.[26] Another study found that the addition of a late afternoon dose of methylphenidate did not significantly alter sleep latency and improved alertness at morning awakening.[29] Another study compared extended-release methylphenidate to dexamphetamine and found that both disturbed sleep and increasing dose was associated with increased sleep disturbance.[26]

Atomoxetine, a nonstimulant drug approved for the treatment of children with ADHD, does not cause insomnia[30,31] or other side effects associated with stimulants. Another study found that methylphenidate increased sleep latency in children with ADHD but that atomoxetine did not.[32]

Because of the insomnia associated with ADHD, one study attempted to treat it with zolpidem. This study reported no effects on polysomnographic recordings including no reduction in sleep latency after 4 weeks of zolpidem administration.[33] A study of melatonin as a treatment for sleep-onset insomnia in children with ADHD found 93% efficacy with short-term melatonin treatment (6 months) and 88% efficacy in the children who continued to use it 3.7 years later.[34]

ADENOTONSILLECTOMY AS TREATMENT FOR ATTENTION DEFICIT/HYPERACTIVITY DISORDER

Unlike the other sections of this article, the beneficial effects of adenotonsillectomy for symptom improvement in children with ADHD are consistent with multiple publications replicating this finding.

In one study, 66 school-age children with ADHD, a polysomnographic diagnosis of mild (AHI <1, >5), and normal to hypertrophic tonsils were compared with 20 normal controls. After evaluation by the ear, nose, and throat department, parents and referring physicians could select treatment of ADHD with methylphenidate, treatment of sleep-disordered breathing with adenotonsillectomy, or no treatment. All children had pre- and postclinical evaluation by a pediatrician, a neurologist, and a psychiatrist. Additionally, they had pre- and post-neurocognitive evaluation; PSG; ADHD rating scale, Child Behavior Checklist (CBCL) filled out by parents and teacher; Test of Variables of Attention (TOVA); and the Quality of Life in Children with Obstructive Sleep Disorder Questionnaire (OSA-18). Twenty-seven of the patients were treated with adenotonsillectomy, 25 with methylphenidate, and 14 had no treatment. The surgical and methylphenidate groups improved more than the nontreatment group. Comparing methylphenidate with adenotonsillectomy, surgery patients had greater improvements in sleep variables, attention span, impulse control, and total ADHD symptoms. The ADHD improvements were statistically significant after surgery and close to normal controls.[35]

The authors suggest that adenotonsillectomy in children with ADHD and mild symptoms of sleep-disordered breathing is of superior efficacy then stimulants and avoids exposing the child to the risks and side effects of this class of drugs. The cause of the symptoms is being addressed rather than controlling the symptoms with medication.

The findings of this study have been replicated by other studies.[13,36,37] One study compared normal-weight children with obese children with ADHD who underwent adenotonsillectomy for OSA. After surgery, all children had improvements in AHI, quality of life, and behavior. Obese children were more likely to have persistent OSA and poor quality of life scores after surgery. Behavior improved postoperatively to a similar extent in all children regardless of obesity.[38]

SUMMARY

Some of our basic assumptions about ADHD in children and sleep are not conclusively supported by sufficient research. Statements made by expert sources are not backed up by conclusive research findings. Although it seems clear that acute sleep deprivation leads to hyperactivity and inattention, it is unclear that children with hyperactivity or inattention have disrupted sleep. Parents of children with ADHD consistently report more bedtime resistance, but there is no consistency in evidence that sleep is subsequently disrupted as measured by actigraphy or polysomnography.

Treatment of ADHD with stimulants may disrupt sleep. Escalating dose or administering an afternoon dose may or may not disrupt sleep. Studies of comorbid sleep disorders such as OSA or PLMs consistently show that they disrupt sleep. Psychiatric disorders that may be present with ADHD in children show that the comorbid psychiatric disorder is associated with disrupted sleep but frequently the control group of ADHD alone sleeps the same as normal controls.

Atomoxetine seems to be superior to stimulant medications in avoiding the risk of sleep disruption. Zolpidem is ineffective in treating sleep problems in children with ADHD. Melatonin, as described in one publication, is an effective treatment of sleep problems in children with ADHD and has demonstrated long-term efficacy.

Clearly, treatment of ADHD in children with mild OSA, that is, an AHI greater than 1, has a beneficial effect that is greater than the effect of stimulant medications and does not have the baggage of side effects that accompany this class of drugs.

The nonmedical literature on children with ADHD suffers from a lack of investigation of sleep issues. Before any child is placed on stimulants, the pediatrician or other health care professional should insure that the child is obtaining adequate sleep and that the parents understand the significance of sleep in avoiding behavioral and psychological symptoms associated with ADHD.

Finally, before a pediatrician places any child on a stimulant medication for ADHD, he or she should carefully question the child's parents about snoring or any sounds of obstructive respiration. The physician must then conduct an airway examination looking not only for hypertrophic tonsils but also the patency of the airway and the possible presence of a large neck or redundant fatty tissue.

Our children's caretakers have a responsibility to insure that children are sleeping adequately and that they do not have mild sleep-disordered breathing before placing a child too young to consent on stimulants.

REFERENCES

1. Gruber R, Wiebe S, Montecalvo L, et al. Effect of sleep restriction on ADHD. Sleep 2011;34(3): 315–23.
2. Available at: http://www.sleepfoundation.org/article/sleep-america-polls/2004-children-and-sleep. Accessed February 14, 2013.
3. Cortese S, Faraone SV, Konofal E, et al. Sleep in children with attention-deficit/hyperactivity disorder: meta-analysis of subjective and objective studies. J Am Acad Child Adolesc Psychiatry 2009;48(9): 894–908.
4. Sadeh A, Pergamin L, Bar-Haim Y. Sleep in children with attention-deficit hyperactivity disorder: a meta-analysis of polysomnographic studies. Sleep Med Rev 2006;10(6):381–98.

5. Hvolby A, Jørgensen J, Bilenberg N. Parental rating of sleep in children with attention deficit/hyperactivity disorder. Eur Child Adolesc Psychiatry 2009;7:429–38.

6. Wiggs L, Montgomery P, Stores G. Actigraphic and parent reports of sleep patterns and sleep disorders in children with subtypes of attention-deficit hyperactivity disorder. Sleep 2005;28(1):1437–45.

7. Corkum P, Tannock R, Moldofsky H, et al. Actigraphy and parental ratings of sleep in children with attention-deficit/hyperactivity disorder (ADHD). Sleep 2001;24(3):303–12.

8. Sangal RB, Owens JA, Sangal J. Patients with attention-deficit/hyperactivity disorder without observed apneic episodes in sleep or daytime sleepiness have normal sleep on polysomnography. Sleep 2005;28(9):1143–8.

9. Hansen BH, Skirbekk B, Oerbeck B, et al. Associations between sleep problems and attentional and behavioral functioning in children with anxiety disorders and ADHD. Behav Sleep Med 2014;12(1):53–68.

10. Chervin RD, Ruzicka DL, Archbold KH, et al. Snoring predicts hyperactivity four years later. Sleep 2005;28(7):885–90.

11. Urschitz MS, Eitner S, Guenther A, et al. Habitual snoring, intermittent hypoxia, and impaired behavior in primary school children. Pediatrics 2004;114(4):1041–8.

12. Chervin RD, Dillon JE, Bassetti C, et al. Symptoms of sleep disorders, inattention, and hyperactivity in children. Sleep 1997;20(12):1185–92.

13. Galland BC, Tripp EG, Gray A, et al. Apnea-hypopnea indices and snoring in children diagnosed with ADHD: a matched case-control study. Sleep Breath 2011;15(3):455–62.

14. Crabtree VM, Ivanenko A, O'Brien LM, et al. Periodic limb movement disorder of sleep in children. J Sleep Res 2003;12(1):73–81.

15. Picchietti DL, England SJ, Walters AS, et al. Periodic limb movement disorder and restless legs syndrome in children with attention-deficit hyperactivity disorder. J Child Neurol 1998;13(12):588–94.

16. Available at: http://www.sleepfoundation.org/article/sleep-topics/adhd-and-sleep. Accessed February 15, 2013.

17. Golan N, Shahar E, Ravid S, et al. Sleep disorders and daytime sleepiness in children with attention-deficit/hyperactive disorder. Sleep 2004;27(2):261–6.

18. Prihodova I, Paclt I, Kemlink D, et al. Sleep disorders and daytime sleepiness in children with attention-deficit/hyperactivity disorder: a two-night polysomnographic study with a multiple sleep latency test. Sleep Med 2010;11(9):922–8.

19. Chiang HL, Gau SS, Ni HC, et al. Association between symptoms and subtypes of attention-deficit hyperactivity disorder and sleep problems/disorders. J Sleep Res 2010;4:535–45.

20. Calhoun SL, Fernandez-Mendoza J, Vgontzas AN, et al. Learning, attention/hyperactivity, and conduct problems as sequelae of excessive daytime sleepiness in a general population study of young children. Sleep 2012;35(5):627–32.

21. Fallone G, Acebo C, Seifer R, et al. Experimental restriction of sleep opportunity in children: effects on teacher ratings. Sleep 2005;28(12):1561–7.

22. Fallone G, Acebo C, Arnedt JT, et al. Effects of acute sleep restriction on behavior, sustained attention, and response inhibition in children. Percept Mot Skills 2001;93(1):213–29.

23. Mayes SD, Calhoun SL, Bixler EO, et al. ADHD subtypes and comorbid anxiety, depression, and oppositional-defiant disorder: differences in sleep problems. J Pediatr Psychol 2009;34(3):328–37.

24. Accardo JA, Marcus CL, Leonard MB, et al. Associations between psychiatric comorbidities and sleep disturbances in children with attention-deficit/hyperactivity disorder. J Dev Behav Pediatr 2012;33(2):97–105.

25. Simonoff E, Taylor E, Baird G. Randomized controlled double-blind trial of optimal dose methylphenidate in children and adolescents with severe attention deficit hyperactivity disorder and intellectual disability. J Child Psychol Psychiatry 2013;54(5):527–35.

26. Stein MA, Waldman ID, Charney E, et al. Dose effects and comparative effectiveness of extended release dexmethylphenidate and mixed amphetamine salts. J Child Adolesc Psychopharmacol 2011;21(6):581–8.

27. Tirosh E, Sadeh A, Munvez R, et al. Effects of methylphenidate on sleep in children with attention-deficient hyperactivity disorder. An activity monitor study. Am J Dis Child 1993;147(12):1313–5.

28. Meijer WM, Faber A, van den Ban E, et al. Current issues around the pharmacotherapy of ADHD in children and adults. Pharm World Sci 2009;31(5):509–16.

29. Kent JD, Blader JC, Koplewicz HS, et al. Effects of late-afternoon methylphenidate administration on behavior and sleep in attention-deficit hyperactivity disorder. Pediatrics 1995;96(2 Pt 1):320–5.

30. Garnock-Jones KP, Keating GM. Atomoxetine: a review of its use in attention-deficit hyperactivity disorder in children and adolescents. Paediatr Drugs 2009;11(3):203–26.

31. Prasad S, Steer C. Switching from neurostimulant therapy to atomoxetine in children and adolescents with attention-deficit hyperactivity disorder: clinical approaches and review of current available evidence. Paediatr Drugs 2008;10(1):39–47.

32. Sangal RB, Owens J, Allen AJ, et al. Effects of atomoxetine and methylphenidate on sleep in children with ADHD. Sleep 2006;29(12):1573–85.

33. Blumer JL, Findling RL, Shih WJ, et al. Controlled clinical trial of zolpidem for the treatment of insomnia associated with attention-deficit/hyperactivity disorder in children 6 to 17 years of age. Pediatrics 2009;123(5):e770–6.

34. Hoebert M, van der Heijden KB, van Geijlswijk IM, et al. Long-term follow-up of melatonin treatment in children with ADHD and chronic sleep onset insomnia. J Pineal Res 2009;47(1):1–7.

35. Huang YS, Guilleminault C, Li HY, et al. Attention-deficit/hyperactivity disorder with obstructive sleep apnea: a treatment outcome study. Sleep Med 2007;8(1):18–30.

36. Wei JL, Bond J, Mayo MS, et al. Improved behavior and sleep after adenotonsillectomy in children with sleep-disordered breathing: long-term follow-up. Arch Otolaryngol Head Neck Surg 2009;135(7): 642–6.

37. Chervin RD, Ruzicka DL, Giordani BJ, et al. Sleep-disordered breathing, behavior, and cognition in children before and after adenotonsillectomy. Pediatrics 2006;117(4):e769–78.

38. Mitchell RB, Boss EF. Pediatric obstructive sleep apnea in obese and normal-weight children: impact of adenotonsillectomy on quality-of-life and behavior. Dev Neuropsychol 2009;34(5):650–61.

Kleine-Levin Syndrome

Isabelle Arnulf, MD, PhD*

KEYWORDS

- Klein-Levin syndrome • Derealization • Recurrent hypersomnia • Hyperphagia

KEY POINTS

- Kleine-Levin syndrome (KLS) is a rare, remittent-relapsing disease mostly affecting adolescents. This syndrome is characterized by episodes of major hypersomnia of one to several weeks, plus cognitive, behavioral, and psychiatric disturbances. Patients are normal between episodes.
- The sudden, severe (more than 18 hours of sleep per day), and recurrent hypersomnia helps differentiating this disease from other psychiatric mimics.
- Despite the fact that hypersexuality, megaphagia, male sex, and teenage onset have been considered as typical features of the disease in some case reports, large series now show a more accurate and different picture, highlighting derealization (a striking feeling of unreality), confusion, and apathy in all patients, while deinhibited behavior is less frequent.
- The disease affect 30%–34% women and 66%–70% men, and child (aged less than 12 years) and adult (aged greater than 20 years) onset has been observed in 10% of the series.
- Episodes tend to be less frequent and tend to disappear with advancing age, with lower sleep quantities. However, one-fourth of patients have long (>30 days) episodes and around 15% have no sign of recovery after more than 20 years of disease.
- Functional brain imaging, during and between episodes, is more useful than sleep monitoring to support the diagnosis.

EPIDEMIOLOGY

The precise prevalence of KLS is unknown, but it is considered a rare disease. In France, the author's experience at a national reference center suggests an estimate of 2.3 cases per million inhabitants.[1] The sex ratio varies from 1/3 to 1/4. Most patients are teenagers during KLS onset, but there are rare cases of onset at around 9 years[2] or after 35 years.[3] The syndrome has been reported worldwide, in Europe, America, Asia, Australia, and Africa. As it is more frequent in Israel,[2,4] and in American Jews,[5] a founding effect is suspected. Although familial risk is low (1% per first-degree relative), there are 5% multiplex families (with brother and sister, parent and child, and cousins),[1,6–9] leading to an estimate of an 800- to 4000-fold increased risk in first-degree relatives.[5]

SYMPTOMS

KLS belongs to the group of recurrent hypersomnia. The diagnosis criteria defined in 2005 are shown in **Box 1**.[10] The first episode usually begins within a few hours, with patients becoming extremely tired, generally after an identifiable triggering event, such as a banal infection in most cases (72%), alcohol intake (alone or combined with a sleep deprivation), or a head trauma. The symptomatic periods last 2 days to several weeks and are characterized by hypersomnia, and cognitive, behavioral, and psychological problems (when awake). The symptoms end suddenly (within an hour) or progressively, within a few days, and they alternate with long (eg, months) periods of normal sleep, cognition, mood, and behavior. The nature and frequency of symptoms are indicated in **Table 1**.

Sleep Disorder Unit, National Reference Center for Narcolepsy, Idiopathic Hypersomnia and Kleine Levin syndrome, Inserm U975, Pitié-Salpêtrière Hospital (APHP), Paris 6 University, Paris, France
* Unité des pathologies du sommeil, Hôpital Pitié-Salpêtrière, 47-83 boulevard de l'Hôpital, 75-651 Paris Cedex 13, France.
E-mail address: isabelle.arnufl@psl.aphp.fr

Sleep Med Clin 10 (2015) 151–161
http://dx.doi.org/10.1016/j.jsmc.2015.02.001
1556-407X/15/$ – see front matter © 2015 Published by Elsevier Inc.

> **Box 1**
> **Diagnosis criteria for Kleine-Levin syndrome**
>
> Kleine-Levin syndrome is defined by the presence of all the following criteria:
>
> A. The patient experiences recurrent episodes of 2 days to several weeks duration, with severe sleepiness.
>
> B. Episodes recur usually more than once a year and at least once every 18 months.
>
> C. The patient has normal alertness, cognitive function, behavior, and mood between episodes,
>
> D. Patients must demonstrate at least one of the following during episodes: cognitive dysfunction, altered perception (mostly derealization), eating disorder (anorexia or hyperphagia), disinhibition (such as hypersexuality)
>
> E. The symptoms are not better explained by another sleep disorder, depression, or bipolar disorder; the effects of medications or drugs; metabolic disorders; or other neurologic, medical, or mental disorders.
>
> *From* American Academy of Sleep Medicine. The International classification of sleep disorders, 3rd edition. Darien (IL): American Academy of Sleep Medicine; 2014; with permission.

Hypersomnia

Teenagers experience a sudden extreme fatigue and a need to rest; they retreat to their rooms and sleep for 15 to 24 h/d, for one to several weeks. The average time asleep per 24 hours is 18 ± 4 hours, with a minimum of 15 ± 5 hours and a maximum of 21 ± 3 hours.[5] Patients remain rousable, but look exhausted and irritable when prevented from sleeping. These long sleep periods may occur night and day, with circadian rhythms exceeding 24 h and possible awakening during the night. Most patients experience intense dreaming and hypnagogic hallucinations (50%), although sleep paralysis is uncommon. Some patients mention that the quality of their dreams changes during the episode, being more frequent (eg, remembering 12 dreams in the same night) and seeming more real than the reality awake. At the end of an episode, most patients experience a transient insomnia. After several episodes, they may not sleep that much but may still need to stay inactive and in the dark, in their room. Typically, the sleep and vigilance are normal between the episodes, when monitored and on questionnaires.

Table 1
Symptoms during at least one KLS episode in a prospective, cross-sectional cohort of 108 patients

Neurologic Symptoms		Psychiatric Symptoms	
Sleep		*Odd behavior*	
Hypersomnia	100%	Hyperphagia	66%
Postepisode transient insomnia	72%	Eat less	34%
Altered cognition	100%	Sexual deinhibition	53%
Slowness (speaking)	94%	Decreased sexuality	6%
Confusion (time > space)	87%	Rudeness	47%
Postepisode amnesia	87%	Compulsive behavior	36%
Apathy	100%	*Psychological problems*	
Altered perception	100%	Depressive mood	53%
Feeling of unreality, dreamy state	81%	Anxiety	45%
Photophobia	59%	Hallucinations	27%
Headache	48%	Delusions	35%

Data from Arnulf I, Lin L, Gadoth N, et al. Kleine-Levin syndrome: a systematic study of 108 patients. Ann Neurol 2008;63:482–93.

Cognitive Impairment

Patients report difficulties to communicate, speak, read, concentrate, decide, memorize, perform 2 tasks simultaneously, coordinate movement, and orientate in time and space (**Fig. 1**). The confusion is, however, mild, and patients continue to be able to count and answer complex questions, but with a slowness that contrasts with their previous cognition. Patients read without understanding what they read, or have difficulty in manipulating the keys of their cell phone. However, despite this feeling of difficulty to coordinate their movement and impaired sensations, there is no ataxia; no motor, sensory, or cranial nerve abnormality, no optic ataxia; and no astereognosia. A neuropsychological test is difficult to perform during the episodes, with patients being very slow and unmotivated. Postepisode partial or complete amnesia is frequent.

The apathy is major and affects all patients. In sharp contrast with their usual teenager concerns, they stop using their cell phone, sending short messages, answering phone calls, playing video games, seeing their friends, smoking, using make

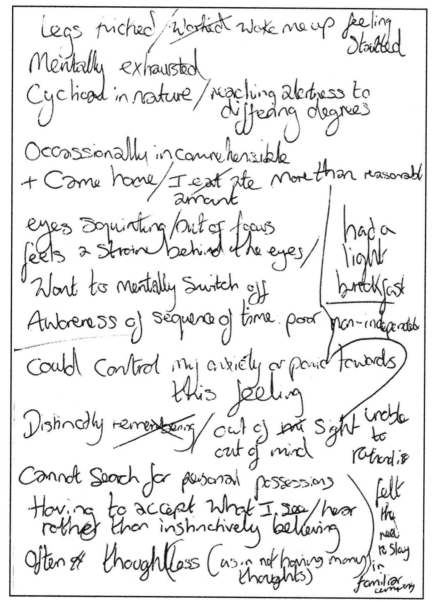

Fig. 1. Symptoms as described by a 19-y-old boy during a KLS episode. Note the incoherent and occasional wrong writing.

up or hair gel, or taking bath or shower. Even speaking seems an effort for them. Patients perform tasks mechanically, as if there were automats. One patient had a KLS episode when skiing. Instead of jumping, skiing fast, and taking risks as he did the previous years, he followed mechanically his brother for 1 week. Another one drove, following the car in front of him for several hours to the point of crossing the France-Belgium border without realizing it, and eventually crashed with a complete amnesia. When seen by clinicians during an episode, patients look exhausted, sleeping, or keeping the eyes closed, totally unconcerned by the medical interview. The interview of the family is much more informative in this case than the patient's interview and examination.

Derealization

Derealization is a clear symptom reported by patients themselves; their perception is altered, resulting in a striking feeling of derealization in all patients. Seeing, hearing, smelling, tasting, feeling cold or hot, and pain could be "wrong." As many as 81% patients feel like being in a dream, as if they were in a vacuum or a bubble, observing the scene from a distant (sometimes upper) perspective, or with a mind-body disconnection. This feeling, occurring at the first minute of the episode, is highly disagreeable and leads some of them to test their environment, that is, break a cup to see if it would break to reassure them that things are normal.

Odd Behavior

The most demonstrative abnormal behaviors in KLS are hyperphagia and hypersexuality. As Critchley[11] was convinced 50 years ago that "morbid hunger" and male sex should be mandatory for the diagnosis of KLS, hyperphagia was reported in 82% of the published cases.[12] After the publication in 2005 of the international KLS criteria, and a systematic interview of more than 100 patients, the megaphagia appears less frequent, in contrast to consistent hypersomnia, cognitive problems, apathy, and derealization. Two-thirds of patients eat more, sometimes compulsively, and eat more sweets and snacks than usual, during some (but not all) of their episodes. The hyperphagia is different from bulimia, because there is no voluntary vomiting or attempt to control weight. Rather, patients are deinhibited toward food, to the point of sometimes stealing candies in their friend's bag or eating all foods in view. Some have fixations on specific food, such as demanding sushi or orange juice. The other one-third of the patients eat rather less: they sleep all the time and are called to the family table, where they eat mechanically. Boys are more often hypersexual than girls (58% vs 35%), with more frequent masturbation (to the point of bleeding, said one) or demand on their sexual partner and inappropriate sexual behaviors, including exposing or touching oneself, masturbating in the presence of parents and clinicians, swearing profanities, touching the nurse's breast, and making inappropriate proposals. Repetitive behaviors are frequent. Around one-third of patients sing singsong, pace, tap, snap fingers, listen to the same music, or watch the same video in a continuous loop. Some patients are in a regressive behavior such as skipping all the time and playing with one's fingers.

Psychiatric Problems

Flattened affect and sad mood (with rare cases of suicidal attempts) are more prevalent in women than in men.[5,13,14] Decreased mood may last only 1 day (often close to the end of an episode), with teenagers crying and feeling that the disease would never end. Some of them clearly ask if they could die from it or would express the desire to die if it does not stop. In rare cases, the sad mood overshoots the sleep episode. Most commonly, the termination of an episode is characterized by a deep feeling of relief, logorrhea, elation, and insomnia, for 1 or 2 days, as if patients would try to make up for the lost time. Anxiety can be high during episodes, with the fear of being left alone at home (and even more in hospital) and of going outside and crossing people (with the shame of crossing strangers, feeling of hostile environment, and even some reference ideas). Some parents describe a regressive behavior, with teenagers speaking with a child voice, using child words, taking a teddy bear, or asking their mothers to sleep near them. On the contrary, some young patients become rude and aggressive, especially when prevented from resting. A child beat his grandmother, an adult patient beat his dog,[15] another child bit his father, a teenager spat on the face of his physician,[16] while a teenager had such an anger outburst at school that the police evacuated the classroom.[17] In one-third of patients, mild, short-lasting hallucinations (a snake near the bed, a dangerous man with a bear in the hospital lift) and delusions are described. Some teenagers affirm to be able to guess the identity of the caller when the phone rings or to stop the clock by thought, have the feeling of having realized the movie that they are looking at, say to the teacher that their (alive) father is dead, have the feeling of being consistently observed or of being poisoned, take themselves for God, or have voices telling them to kill their father. The delusional episode is usually short, lasting a few hours to a few days, and stops spontaneously. All these psychological symptoms contrast dramatically with the usual behavior and psychological profile of the teenager.

Autonomic Symptoms

Headache, photophobia, phonophobia, and sweating are frequent. The teenager's face during the episode is usually tired, with an empty gaze and possibly flushing. Patients may void less often (eg, only once a day), and have, in rare cases, urine retention. Other autonomic signs are exceptional, including abnormally high or low blood pressure,[18] bradycardia or tachycardia,[3] and ataxic respiration.

CLINICAL FORMS

Despite KLS being a rare disease, it is possible to observe various forms of the disease. Contrary to ancient small series, the full-blown KLS does not mandatorily include the hypersomnia plus hyperphagia plus hypersexuality triad (which is present in only 45% patients), but rather the hypersomnia plus confusion plus apathy plus derealization tetrad, which is found in 100% patients.[1,5]

There are some mild, benign forms of KLS, with teenagers experiencing 1-week symptomatic periods 2 to 3 times a year. In contrast, some patients experience 7- to 10-day episodes every month, whereas others have long-lasting (eg, 3–6 months) episodes with an altered cognition, apathy, and sleep cycling on rhythm greater than 24 hours. Up to one-third of the patients have prolonged (greater than 1 month) episodes.[1] Eventually, some patients may experience 40 to 80 episodes with no evidence of cure, and possibly a long-term alteration of attention or mood.[19,20] When KLS starts after the age of 20 years, the chance of spontaneous disappearance of the disease is much lower. All in all, the former concept of a benign disease that spontaneously disappears should now be challenged.

Secondary KLS, observed in 10% patients,[1,21] is one in which neurologic symptoms are present before KLS onset and persists between episodes. KLS-like symptoms have been observed in association with stroke or posttraumatic brain hematoma, genetic or developmental diseases (including mosaicism, Prader-Willi syndrome, Asperger syndrome, mental retardation), multiple sclerosis, hydrocephalus, paraneoplasia, autoimmune encephalitis, and severe infectious encephalitis.

Menstruation-linked hypersomnia[22] resembles KLS, with hypersomnia behavioral, cognitive, and mood problems being timely associated with menstruation (just before or at the time of) and even puerperium,[12] and it is now considered a form of KLS.[23]

Recently, some investigators have described patients with recurrent, sudden-onset/offset episodes with slowed cognition, derealization, and hyperphagia, which were not associated with hypersomnia but with insomnia.[24] Similarly, the author has seen a teenager with all KLS symptoms but normal sleep during 7 discrete episodes of 10 days. As sleep may be shortened or normal during some episodes (especially during the last ones) in patients with otherwise typical KLS, the author suspects that these patients have borderline forms of KLS, with symptoms varying with function of the brain area affected by the encephalitis.

EVOLUTION OF THE DISEASE
Duration and Frequency of Episodes

The episodes follow an unpredictable course. Episodes last a mean of 13 days, but miniepisodes lasting 1 to 2 days (generally during a week-end) may occur between long episodes. On the other hand, very long (3–4 months) episodes are observed in rare but otherwise typical KLS cases.[1,6] During a given episode, the hypersomnia is generally marked during the first days, and changes toward less sleep and more apathy and altered cognition at the end of the episode. After several episodes, the symptoms may change, with episodes containing less sleep and more apathy and altered cognition. The mean interval between episodes is 5.7 months, with ranges of 0.5 to 66 months. Episodes recur more frequently in patients with childhood onset. Patients have an average of 19 episodes.

Disease Duration

In the author's prospective series of 108 patients, the disease lasts a median of 13.6 ± 4.3 years. It is therefore common to say to the patient and the family that the disease will disappear (in most cases) after the age of 30 years. Male sex and presence of hypersexuality are associated with longer disease duration. When KLS starts after the age of 20 years, it is not possible to calculate the disease course, because more than 50% of the patients with KLS are not cured after 25 years, suggesting that the disease is more fixed in the adult-onset form.[5] In the meta-analysis of 186 KLS cases in the literature, patients with numerous episodes during the first year of the disease had shorter course.[21]

DIFFERENTIAL DIAGNOSIS
Organic Diagnoses

As the disease is exceptional and not known from many practitioners, several more common diseases are usually evoked first (**Table 2**). When

Table 2
Differential diagnoses of KLS

Disease	Differential Features and Tests	Episodic
Intoxication with		
Cannabis, drugs	Urine screen for toxic	Yes
Alcohol	Alcohol blood levels	Yes
Benzodiazepines	Urine screen for toxic	Yes
Periodic hypersomnias[a]		
Idiopathic recurrent stupor	EEG, CSF screening, flumazenil challenge	Always
Menstruation-linked hypersomnia	Always associated with the menstruations; therapeutic challenge with a contraceptive blocking the hormonal axis	Always
Metabolic diseases		
Hyperammonemic encephalitis	Ammonemia	Yes
Intermittent porphyria		
Neurologic diseases		
Temporal partial seizure	EEG, long-term EEG	Yes
Brain frontal/temporal lesion (tumor, inflammation, stroke, hematoma)	Brain MRI	Yes (inflammation)
Basilar migraine	Short (24–48 h) hypersomnia episodes, headaches	Yes
Meningoencephalitis	Fever, spinal tap (increased white blood cells and protein levels in CSF), check for Lyme serology	No
Lewy body dementia	Intermittent vigilance and cognition fluctuation in a patient *older than 50 y*; screen for memory defect, parkinsonism, and REM sleep behavior disorder	Frequently
Klüver-Bucy syndrome	Brain MRI	No
Psychiatric diseases	In general, no confusion; symptomatic EEG gives normal result	
Psychosis	Depersonnalization/derealization Hallucinations, delusions	Rarely
Bipolar disease	Depressive and manic episodes are *longer* (months) than KLS episodes, and not associated with confusion	Yes
Depression with atypical features	Decreased mood may be associated with hypersomnia	
Seasonal affective disorder	Prolonged depression, anergy, hypersomnia, hyperphagia, weight gain, sweet craving, and loss of concentration occur during autumn/ winter	Yes
Crepuscular state in conversion neurosis	Episodes of pseudoconfusion are short (<24 h)	Yes

Abbreviations: CSF, cerebrospinal fluid; EEG, electroencephalography.
[a] Excessive sleepiness in sleep apnea, narcolepsy, and idiopathic hypersomnia is not recurrent but consistent.

brought to the emergency department during the first episodes, before the KLS diagnosis is performed, most patients undergo the classic tests in case of sudden confusion and behavioral changes in teenagers. These tests include checking for alcohol as well as drug and illegal substance intake; performing brain morphologic imaging (mostly an MRI) for ruling out tumor, inflammatory disease, multiple sclerosis, and stroke; performing electroencephalography (EEG) to detect temporal status epilepticus; measuring serum levels of ammonia for hyperammonemic encephalitis, testing for intermittent porphyria and Lyme disease, and frequently, performing a spinal tap looking for encephalitis (mandatory if fever is present). All these tests usually give normal results in KLS, although a few, nonspecific EEG sharp waves may be observed. Among these tests, EEG is the most helpful, because it documents localized or generalized background slowing in up to 70% of the patients with KLS during an episode (see **Fig. 3**). Several symptoms, such as food utilization, verbal perseverations, withdrawal, and deinhibited behavior, remind of frontal lobe syndrome, while the association of megaphagia and hypersexuality has also been described in Klüver-Bucy syndrome associated with bitemporal lesions and in orbitofrontal lesions. In contrast to KLS, symptoms are continuous and not intermittent in these syndromes. Idiopathic stupor is a rare and debated differential diagnosis of KLS, occurring usually in middle-aged subjects, with stuporous episodes lasting no more than 48 h.

Psychiatric Diagnoses

Many patients are referred to child or adult psychiatric departments before the diagnosis of KLS is made. The main differences between KLS with psychotic symptoms and psychotic disorders are the sudden aspect of delusion and hallucinations in KLS, the absence of long-term adhesion to the belief, the presence of associated neurologic symptoms (mainly slowness, confusion, amnesia, and hypersomnia), and the abrupt cessation of the psychotic symptoms. The recurrence of symptoms after one to several months without psychosis is also characteristic of KLS. The difference between KLS with mood changes and a depressive disorder is how suddenly the symptoms come and then go, in a previously happy teenager, and their association with cognitive and behavioral symptoms. A teenager sleeping more than 20 hours a day is also uncommon in depressive disorders, even when severe. Also, an abnormal result of EEG, with slow waves when awake, suggests an organic disorder.

TESTS
Brain Imaging

Results of morphologic brain imaging (computed tomography, MRI) are normal, except for unspecific variants of the norms. Functional brain imaging (single-photon emission computed tomography [SPECT]) documents several areas of hypoperfusion during the episodes (thalamus, hypothalamus, as well as temporal, frontal, and sometimes parietal and occipital areas), which may persist, at a lower degree, in asymptomatic periods[18,25–27] in half of the patients (**Fig. 2**). Specifically, in a group analysis of 41 patients, the parietotemporal junction was hypoperfused during episodes, in proportion with the intensity of derealization, suggesting that this area, which integrates the cross-modal sensorial information, is causing this derealization symptoms.[28]

Electroencephalography

One-fourth of the patients have normal results of EEG during episodes. In 70% of the patients, a nonspecific diffuse slowing of background EEG activity, such as the alpha frequency band being slowed toward 7 to 8 Hz, is observed.[29,30] Less frequently, low-frequency high-amplitude waves (delta or theta) occur in isolation or in sequence, mainly in the bilateral temporal or temporofrontal areas, paralleling the SPECT findings (**Fig. 3**).

Sleep Studies

In the author's experience, sleep monitoring is not very useful for the diagnosis of KLS. It may be difficult to organize sleep monitoring during the first

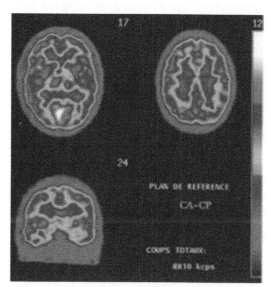

Fig. 2. Brain scintigraphy during a KLS episode in a boy.

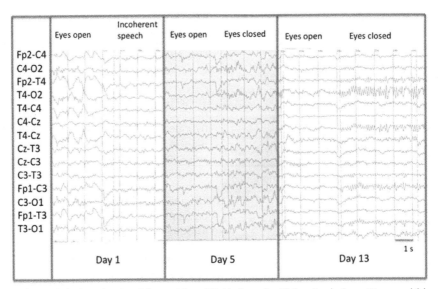

Fig. 3. EEG performed during the 1st, 5th, and last (13th) day of a KLS episode in a 17-year-old boy. Note the diffuse EEG slow waves on day 1 (even when speaking), which prevail on the right hemisphere on day 5 and disappear the last day.

days of an episode because of the following: the sleep duration and structure depend on the time when the test is performed, most patients cannot comply with the multiple sleep latency test procedure (which can contain short sleep onset latencies and sleep onset in rapid eye movement [REM] periods, transiently resembling narcolepsy in one-third to one-sixth of the patients), and they may stay hours in bed in a generalized hypoarousal, with a diffuse alpha EEG rhythm alternating with fragmented sleep stage N1. An example of this is the 24-hour sleep monitoring in an 18-year-old patient at the beginning of a KLS episode. When systematically analyzing the literature, the mean total sleep time was 445 ± 122 min during the night (stage 1, 6 ± 4%; stage 2, 56 ± 9%; stages 3 and 4, 19 ± 11%; REM sleep, 19 ± 6%). Night sleep lasted 568 ± 204 min during an episode and 384 ± 59 min between in a series of 14 patients studied in Israel.[31] In a series of 18 patients monitored for 24 hours while in an episode, the total sleep duration was 701 ± 270 min.[8] In a series of 17 patients in Taiwan, when nighttime sleep was monitored before the end of the first half of the symptomatic period, an important reduction in slow-wave sleep was present with progressive return to normal during the second half despite the persistence of clinical symptoms.[32] REM sleep was normal in the first half of the episode but decreased in the second half.

Biological Markers

There is no biological marker for KLS yet. Serum biology is typically normal during and between

the episode, including inflammation markers and white blood cells. The author has found similar C-reactive protein levels in 108 patients with KLS versus controls.[5] The agents responsible for this first infection, when it triggers KLS, are rarely identified, and include Epstein-Barr virus, varicella virus, Asian influenza virus, enterovirus, H1N1 virus, and streptococcus. The hormonal pituitary axis is normal, except for a few inconsistent abnormalities.[33] Leptin levels are also normal.[5]

As young age of onset, recurrence, and presence of inflammatory lesions in the brain may suggest that KLS is an autoimmune disease, the human leukocyte antigen class II genotypes were studied in 30 European trios with KLS trios, 108 American trios with KLS, and 120 French patients with KLS. There was a twice greater frequency of DRB1*0301-DQB1*0201 and DRB1*0701-DQB1*0202 genotypes in European patients with KLS,[8] an association that was not replicated in the larger American study[5] and in the larger French study,[1] suggesting it was a random result.

Cerebrospinal fluid (CSF) white blood cell count and protein count are normal in patients, ruling out meningitis. There was no oligoclonal secretion of antibodies (as in multiple sclerosis, another remitting neurologic disease) in the CSF of 4 patients with KLS. The CSF levels of hypocretin are within normal ranges, although they can be slightly lower during than between episodes.[6,34,35]

Neuropathology

The examination of brain has been performed after the death of 4 patients (with primary, n = 2, and

Box 2
Suggested management of a patient with KLS

1. Obtain a detailed history from the parents or spouse.

2. Check for normal brain imaging, EEG, and psychiatric examination out of an episode.

3. During the episodes, recommend to let the patient sleep at home, under family supervision. This attitude limits the fear for novelty and the risk of embarrassing public behaviors and is safer for the patient. The attempts to wake up or stimulate the patient are useless, because the disease is an encephalitis.

4. Firmly recommend not to drive a car or a motorbike during an episode, because sleepiness, automatic behavior, and altered perception expose to a high risk of road accident.

5. Recommend the family to regularly check during an episode if the patient drinks and eats enough (in case of reduced drinking and eating) or not too much (in case of hyperphagia), urinates at least once a day (in case of urine retention), and has no suicidal ideas.

6. Between episodes, keep regular sleep/wake schedules and avoid alcohol and contact with infectious subjects.

7. Try, at least once, amantadine at the beginning of an episode, because it can abort an episode.

8. During an episode, in case of intense anxious symptoms, use sublingual bromazepam. If delusions or behavioral disturbances are severe enough to justify a neuroleptic treatment, consider a very short treatment with risperidone.

9. If episodes are long or frequent (eg, every 1–3 months), consider using prolonged-release lithium (in order to obtain a serum lithium level between 0.8 and 1.2 mmol/L). Reevaluate the benefit/risk ratio every 6 months.

Abbreviation: EEG, electroencephalography.

secondary KLS, n = 2).[36–39] The cortex was intact in 3 patients, while a patient with KLS secondary to a paraneoplastic syndrome had perivascular infiltrates in the amygdala and temporal lobe. There were intense signs of inflammatory encephalitis within the thalamus and hypothalamus in 2 patients (abundant infiltrates of inflammatory cells, perivascular lympho-monocyte infiltrate, microglial proliferation), mild inflammation in one patient, and none in the last patient (only mildly depigmented substantia nigra and locus coeruleus).

MANAGEMENT AND TREATMENT

The author's suggestions are displayed in **Box 2**. Many drug trials have been disappointing in KLS. However, a few drugs may help to manage the symptoms during the episodes and to prevent the recurrence of episodes in between. During the episodes, the usual stimulants (modafinil, methylphenidate, and amphetamine) are rarely beneficial and may at best unmask the other disagreeable cognitive and behavioral symptoms. Amantadine, which is also an antiviral, may curiously help to abort episodes when given since the first day. When psychotic symptoms are prolonged and prominent, risperidone seems more helpful than other neuroleptics. In case of major anxiety, benzodiazepine may help the patients.

The episodes are usually too short to require and benefit from antidepressants drugs.

As for preventing new relapses when the episodes are frequent (ie, occurring 4–12 times/year), daily prevention with lithium may be tried.[21] There is no explanation on how this drug helps in KLS and especially no link (personal and familial) with bipolar disease.[5] The benefit (25%–75%)/risk ratio should be reevaluated every 6 months. The author has had a good experience with lithium therapy in more than 70 patients, with serum lithium levels between 0.8 and 1.2 mmol/L. The antiepileptics (eg, valproate) seem less efficacious in the author's experience (and when looking at all published cases and the author's series). When the episodes are timely associated with menstruations, a blockade of the hypophysis axis with high doses of estroprogestative may be tried. Antidepressants are devoid of prophylactic effects in KLS.

SUMMARY

KLS is an intriguing, severe, and homogenous disease, known for more than a century, with no obvious cause or treatment. Recent methods of investigation such as SPECT indicate that the brain dysfunction is larger than expected, and encompasses both cortical (frontal, internal temporal lobe) and subcortical (and especially thalamus and hypothalamus) areas. In addition, persistent post-KLS memory and SPECT defects recently observed in a few cases raise the possibility of long-term brain damage in a disease that was assumed to be benign. The finding of a possible Jewish predisposition, occasional familial clustering, and the association with infectious triggering factors suggest that KLS is due to environmental factors acting on a vulnerable genetic background. This general picture and the fluctuating symptoms in KLS are consistent with the possibility of an autoimmune mediation of the disorder.

ACKNOWLEDGMENTS

The author thanks the Kleine-Levin Foundation (Boston, USA), which allowed the author's group to start working on this disease and supported their recent study on functional brain imaging in KLS. The French KLS research program is financed by the national grant PHRC 070138 and by the Institut Hospital-Universitaire de Neurosciences of Pitié-Slapêtrière Hospital.

REFERENCES

1. Lavault S, Golmard J, Groos E, et al. Kleine-Levin syndrome in 120 patients: differential diagnosis and long episodes. Ann Neurol 2015;77:529–40.
2. Kesler A, Gadoth N, Vainstein G, et al. Kleine Levin syndrome (KLS) in young females. Sleep 2000;23:563–7.
3. Hegarty A, Merriam AE. Autonomic events in Kleine-Levin syndrome. Am J Psychiatry 1990;147:951–2.
4. Lavie P, Gadoth N, Gordon CR, et al. Sleep patterns in Kleine-Levin syndrome. Electroencephalogr Clin Neurophysiol 1979;47:369–71.
5. Arnulf I, Lin L, Gadoth N, et al. Kleine-Levin syndrome: a systematic study of 108 patients. Ann Neurol 2008;63:482–93.
6. Katz JD, Ropper AH. Familial Kleine-Levin syndrome: two siblings with unusually long hypersomnic spells. Arch Neurol 2002;59:1959–61.
7. Janicki S, Franco K, Zarko R. A case report of Kleine-Levin syndrome in an adolescent girl. Psychosomatics 2001;42:350–2.
8. Dauvilliers Y, Mayer G, Lecendreux M, et al. Kleine-Levin syndrome: an autoimmune hypothesis based on clinical and genetic analyses. Neurology 2002;59:1739–45.
9. Bahammam A, Gadelrab M, Owais S, et al. Clinical characteristics and HLA typing of a family with Kleine-Levin syndrome. Sleep Med 2008;9:575–8.
10. American Academy of Sleep Medicine. The International classification of sleep disorders - revised. In: Hauri P, editor. Chicago: American Academy of Sleep Medicine; 2005. p. 1–297.
11. Critchley M. Periodic hypersomnia and megaphagia in adolescent males. Brain 1962;85:627–56.
12. Billiard M, Jaussent I, Dauvilliers Y, et al. Recurrent hypersomnia: a review of 339 cases. Sleep Med Rev 2011;15:247–57.
13. Gallinek A. The Kleine-Levin syndrome: hypersomnia, bulimia, and abnormal mental states. World Neurol 1962;3:235–43.
14. Vlach V. Periodical somnolence, bulimia and mental changes (Kleine-Levin Syndrome). Cesk Neurol 1962;25:401–5.
15. Yassa R, Nair NP. The Kleine-Levine syndrome–a variant? J Clin Psychiatry 1978;39:254–9.
16. Mukaddes NM, Kora ME, Bilge S. Carbamazepine for Kleine-Levin syndrome. J Am Acad Child Adolesc Psychiatry 1999;38:791–2.
17. Crumley FE. Valproic acid for Kleine-Levin syndrome. J Am Acad Child Adolesc Psychiatry 1997;36:868–9.
18. Portilla P, Durand E, Chalvon A, et al. SPECT-identified hypoperfusion of the left temporomesial structures in a Kleine-Levin syndrome. Rev Neurol (Paris) 2002;158:593–5 [in French].
19. Landtblom AM, Dige N, Schwerdt K, et al. Short-term memory dysfunction in Kleine-Levin syndrome. Acta Neurol Scand 2003;108:363–7.
20. Engström M, Vigren P, Karlsson T, et al. Working memory in 8 Kleine-Levin syndrome patients: an fMRI study. Sleep 2009;32:681–8.
21. Arnulf I, Zeitzer JM, File J, et al. Kleine-Levin syndrome: a systematic review of 186 cases in the literature. Brain 2005;128:2763–76.
22. Billiard M, Guilleminault C, Dement WC. A menstruation-linked periodic hypersomnia. Kleine-Levin syndrome or new clinical entity? Neurology 1975;25:436–43.
23. American Academy of Sleep Medicine. The International classification of sleep disorders. 3rd edition. Darien (IL): American Academy of Sleep Medicine; 2014.
24. Shukla G, Bhatia M, Singh S, et al. Atypical Kleine-Levin syndrome: can insomnia and anorexia be features too? Sleep Med 2008;9:172–6.
25. Landtblom AM, Dige N, Schwerdt K, et al. A case of Kleine-Levin syndrome examined with SPECT and neuropsychological testing. Acta Neurol Scand 2002;105:318–21.
26. Lu ML, Liu HC, Chen CH, et al. Kleine-Levin syndrome and psychosis: observation from an unusual case. Neuropsychiatry Neuropsychol Behav Neurol 2000;13:140–2.
27. Huang YS, Guilleminault C, Kao PF, et al. SPECT findings in the Kleine-Levin syndrome. Sleep 2005;28:955–60.
28. Kas A, Lavault S, Habert MO, et al. Feeling unreal: a functional imaging study in 41 patients with Kleine-Levin syndrome. Brain 2014;137:2077–87.

29. Vollmer R, Toifl K, Kothbauer P, et al. EEG- and biochemical findings in Kleine-Levin-syndrome. A case report (author's transl). Nervenarzt 1981;52: 211–8 [in German].

30. Papacostas SS, Hadjivasilis V. The Kleine-Levin syndrome. Report of a case and review of the literature. Eur Psychiatry 2000;15:231–5.

31. Gadoth N, Kesler A, Vainstein G, et al. Clinical and polysomnographic characteristics of 34 patients with Kleine-Levin syndrome. J Sleep Res 2001;10: 337–41.

32. Huang Y, Lin Y, Guilleminault C. Polysomnography in Kleine-Levin syndrome. Neurology 2008;70: 795–801.

33. Mayer G, Leonhard E, Krieg J, et al. Endocrinological and polysomnographic findings in Kleine-Levin syndrome: no evidence for hypothalamic and circadian dysfunction. Sleep 1998;21:278–84.

34. Mignot E, Lammers GJ, Ripley B, et al. The role of cerebrospinal fluid hypocretin measurement in the diagnosis of narcolepsy and other hypersomnias. Arch Neurol 2002;59:1553–62.

35. Dauvilliers Y, Baumann CR, Carlander B, et al. CSF hypocretin-1 levels in narcolepsy, Kleine-Levin syndrome, and other hypersomnias and neurological conditions. J Neurol Neurosurg Psychiatry 2003;74: 1667–73.

36. Carpenter S, Yassa R, Ochs R. A pathologic basis for Kleine-Levin syndrome. Arch Neurol 1982;39: 25–8.

37. Koerber RK, Torkelson R, Haven G, et al. Increased cerebrospinal fluid 5-hydroxytryptamine and 5-hydroxyindoleacetic acid in Kleine-Levin syndrome. Neurology 1984;34:1597–600.

38. Takrani LB, Cronin D. Kleine-Levin syndrome in a female patient. Can Psychiatr Assoc J 1976;21:315–8.

39. Fenzi F, Simonati A, Crosato F, et al. Clinical features of Kleine-Levin syndrome with localized encephalitis. Neuropediatrics 1993;24:292–5.

Rapid Eye Movement Sleep Behavior Disorder During Childhood

Suresh Kotagal, MD

KEYWORDS

- Rapid eye movement sleep • Behavior disorder • Childhood • Narcolepsy
- Neurodevelopmental disabilities • Chairi malformation

KEY POINTS

- RBD can occur in childhood, though infrequently.
- Neurodevelopmental disorders, narcolepsy and medication effect are common etiologies.
- In contrast to adult, association with synucleinopathies is not seen.
- Treament may consist of withdrawal of causative medication, eg, selective serotonin reuptake inhibitor, or prescription of melatonin.

INTRODUCTION

In 1987, Schenck and colleagues[1] had described a new type of parasomnia in older men that arose out of rapid eye movement (REM) sleep and was characterized by aggressive or violent motor dream enactment in conjunction with preservation of tonic electromyographic activity (ie, REM sleep without atonia). Subsequently defined as REM sleep behavior disorder (RBD), this parasomnia is now recognized to occur at all ages and in both sexes, although it remains relatively infrequent during childhood. The literature pertaining to RBD in childhood is scant, and composed only of single case reports or small case series. The reasons for why the disorder has been infrequently documented in childhood are unclear; is it being under-recognized by sleep specialists, or is it truly low in occurrence in this age group? In adults, RBD has an association with neurodegenerative disorders termed synucleinopathies. This category of disorders includes Parkinson disease, multi-system atrophy, and dementia with Lewy body disease. Narcolepsy, with or without cataplexy is also associated with RBD in adults, as is the use of certain psychotropic medications. The clinical features of childhood RBD are distinct from the previously described associations of adult RBD, and were discussed by Stores in 2008.[2] An updated review of childhood RBD is presented in this article.

PERSPECTIVE FROM SLEEP ONTOGENESIS

By the time a prematurely born infant has reached 30 to 32 weeks of postconceptional age, there is clear differentiation of sleep into active (REM) and quiet (non-REM [NREM]) categories, with the former constituting about 80% of the total sleep time. Concurrent with neuromaturation, there is progressive reduction in the proportion of REM sleep and a corresponding increase in NREM sleep. A third type of electroencephalographic (EEG) behavioral state (besides REM and NREM sleep) is also seen in premature infants. It is termed transitional sleep, and is composed of admixed elements of both REM and NREM sleep, such as presence of tonic electromyographic

Conflicts of Interest: None.
Funding Source: None.
Division of Child Neurology, Mayo Clinic, 200 First Street, Rochester, MN 55905, USA
E-mail address: Kotagal.suresh@mayo.edu

Sleep Med Clin 10 (2015) 163–167
http://dx.doi.org/10.1016/j.jsmc.2015.02.004

activity in conjunction with low-voltage irregular electroencephalographic activity that is generally observed in REM sleep.[3] Transitional sleep is most common between 34 to 38 weeks postconceptional age and resolves thereafter with cortical maturation. From the standpoint of sleep ontogeny, one could postulate therefore that transitional sleep, when composed of bursts of eye movements, bodily twitches, and tonic chin electromyographic sleep, resembles REM sleep without atonia (RSWA), which could be the hypothetical polysomnographic correlate of RBD in an infant. The appearance of RBD or REM sleep without atonia in childhood/adolescence/adults could thus represent regression to a more primitive, undifferentiated state of sleep.

PREVALENCE

Given that there are few reported studies on childhood RBD, it is hard to determine the exact prevalence of childhood RBD. The nature of the disorder is such that, unlike other childhood parasomnias like sleep terrors, sleep walking, or confusional arousals that can be suspected based upon history, RBD requires nocturnal polysomnography in the sleep laboratory environment for making a diagnosis. Population-based estimates are thus difficult to develop. The semiology does have some resemblance to nightmares, because the individual is experiencing a terrifying dream. Partinen and Hublin found that nightmares occur always or often in 2% to 11% of children, and now and then in 15% to 31% of children.[4]

PATHOPHYSIOLOGY

The key features of RBD on polysomnography are preserved chin electromyographic tone, or RSWA, and video evidence of motor dream enactment in the form of increased physical activity, including aggressive or violent behaviors. These aggressive behaviors may result in injury to self, others, or to property. During RSWA, there is no overt clinical behavioral disturbance but presence of only polygraphic sleep abnormalities. RSWA may occur independent of RBD, but RBD always requires the presence of RSWA. Although it may appear attractive to postulate that RSWA is a biomarker for RBD, there are no longitudinal data to indicate that the former consistently evolves into the latter. RSWA is defined by the American Academy of Sleep Medicine as either short phasic bursts of 0.1 to 14.9 seconds, or as tonic segments of 15 seconds or longer duration, exceeding 2 to 4 times the lowest level background electromyogram (EMG) amplitude, with 5 mini-epochs of

3 second duration within a 30 second epoch of REM sleep.[5] The pathophysiologic mechanisms for RBD have been discussed by Boeve and colleagues.[6] There is dysregulation of inhibitory brainstem motor mechanisms. Although the exact pathway in people has not been determined, neuroimaging data from human RBD cases have implicated the dorsal midbrain and pontine regions. Studies in cats implicate the subcoeruleus region, while rat studies suggest the sublaterodorsal nucleus as being crucial to the pathophysiology of RBD.[6]

In adults, RBD has been categorized into the cryptogenic and secondary or symptomatic forms.[7] The former group is not associated with any overt clinical or neuroimaging abnormalities, but a concern remains whether those diagnosed with cryptogenic RBD will develop a synucleinopathy several years later, and if RBD in this population is a biomarker for neurodegenerative disease. The secondary or symptomatic form of RBD in adults occurs in association with a known synucleinopathy such as dementia with Lewy body disease, idiopathic Parkinson disease, or multisystem atrophy.[6,7] In adults and children, narcolepsy with cataplexy more so than narcolepsy without cataplexy is associated with RBD.[8] It is possible that RBD associated with narcolepsy–cataplexy differs mechanistically from that observed in neurodegenerative disorders, as the former is associated with low cerebrospinal fluid hypocretin levels.[9]

In childhood RBD, there is obviously no association with progressive disturbances of synuclein metabolism, although admittedly neuropathologic studies are completely lacking. From another standpoint, static neurodevelopmental disabilities such as autism, Moebius syndrome, and Smith Magenis syndrome; structural brainstem lesions such as neoplasms or Chiari type 1 malformation; narcolepsy; juvenile Parkinson disease; and the use of psychotropic medications predominate.[10–17] The common link between RBD of childhood and that of adults is the identical final common pathway leading up to event (ie, sleep state dissociation).[18] This is a process whereby elements of wakefulness such as tonic electromyographic activity, vocalizations, and bodily movement become superimposed on the phenomena of REM sleep.

CLINICAL MANIFESTATIONS

Medical or neurologic disorders that have been linked to childhood onset RBD are listed in **Table 1**. There are no overt clinical manifestations of RSWA, as this is solely a polysomnographic finding. Of note, however, it is not known if a

Table 1
Etiology of rapid eye movement sleep behavior disorder in childhood

Category	Disorder
Neurodevelopmental disabilities	Autism[13] Smith Magenis syndrome[21] Moebius syndrome[10]
Structural brainstem lesions	Pontine glioma[10] Chiari malformation type 1[12]
Movement disorders	Juvenile Parkinson disease[11] Tourette syndrome[16]
Primary hypersomnia/ degenerative	Narcolepsy–cataplexy/ narcolepsy[2,8,9]
Medication induced	Selective serotonin reuptake inhibitors such as fluoxetine, venlafaxine, and clomipramine; tricyclic agents; withdrawal of barbiturates, bisoprolol, caffeine, or alcohol[17]

patient who demonstrates RSWA on 1 night's polysomnogram will consistently demonstrate the same finding on a repeat sleep study, or if he or she could, on a subsequent night, manifest overt RBD. This type of longitudinal data has not been reported in children or adolescents. The framework proposed by Schenck and colleagues[19] in 1993 regarding the classification of clinical features of RBD in adults is helpful, and can be applied to childhood cases also. It subdivides the clinical manifestations of RBD into: (1) vocalizations such as yelling, swearing, talking or laughing; (2) mimics or pantomimes of everyday life such as gesturing with hands, sitting, combing hair, or fishing, and (3) aggressive or violent movements such as punching, kicking, aiming.

The age of onset of RBD in childhood can be as early as 2 to 3 years. The presenting symptoms are of 2 types:

1. Those related to RBD itself; these include yelling in REM sleep, moving the arms and legs vigorously, pantomimic behaviors such as gesturing with the hands or actual punching and kicking of bedmate siblings. In a study of 37 adult, drug-naïve narcolepsy–cataplexy related RBD subjects, Cipolli and colleagues[9] felt that violent aggressive behavior was seen less often when RBD occurred during the first half of the night. Similar observations have not been made in childhood-onset RBD. When childhood RBD patients have the capacity to communicate verbally, they may recall a fearful dream that involves the patient or family members being attacked by an intruder (author's unpublished observation, 1996). The duration of the RBD event is generally 0.5 to 2 minutes. There are no definite postictal manifestations. The simultaneously obtained electroencephalogram remains normal.

2. Symptoms from the underlying disorder that is predisposing to RBD (eg, a child with autism may have poor eye contact, an odd speech pattern, prefer to play with toys rather than other children, and exhibit stereotyped hand flapping or toe walking.[20] The patient with Smith Magenis syndrome is aggressive or hyperactive during the daytime, and shows mildly dysmorphic facial features in the form of square-shaped forehead, low-set ears, and brachycephaly.[21] It is related to a microdeletion or mutation in the retinoic acid-induced 1 (*RAI1*) gene. There may be inversion in the pattern of release of melatonin, with low levels at night, and higher levels during the day. Tourette syndrome is characterized by chronic motor and vocal tics of more than 12 months' duration, with a tendency for the tics to fluctuate in severity; comorbid attention deficit disorder and obsessive–compulsive disorder are seen in close to 50% of children.[22] Structural brainstem lesions such as pontine glioma are associated with ipsilateral sixth or seventh cranial nerve palsy in conjunction with contralateral hemiparesis. A symptomatic Chiari type 1 malformation may be accompanied by dysphagia to liquids, paradoxic vocal cord motion on laryngoscopy, central sleep apnea on polysomnography, and MRI evidence of caudal displacement of the cerebellar tonsils in conjunction with brainstem compression.[12] In childhood narcolepsy–cataplexy, RBD may be the initial manifestation.[15] It may be accompanied by hypersomnolence, cataplexy, positive blood test for HLADQB1*0602, and low levels of spinal fluid hypocretin.[15] With regard to medication-induced RBD, such as that related to the use of tricyclic or selective serotonin reuptake inhibitor (SSRI) agents, there may be associated manifestations of the underlying psychiatric disorder.[17]

DIAGNOSIS

The diagnosis of RBD is established on the basis of clinical features combined with characteristic findings on video nocturnal polysomnography. There is presence of RSWA. Further, a review of the video recording shows excessive body movement during REM sleep. It is important to ensure that augmentation of chin electromyographic tone observed on nocturnal polysomnography is not temporally related to obstructive sleep apnea, periodic limb movements, seizures, or gastroesophageal reflux, and misinterpreted as RSWA. The value of additional EMG monitoring from muscles of the forearm in childhood RBD has not been established.

MANAGEMENT

If the patient does not have an underlying neurologic, psychiatric or genetic diagnosis, the disorder is not medication-induced, and RBD and RSWA are incidentally recognized during nocturnal polysomnography, the sleep specialist should refer the patient to a child neurologist or pediatrician, who should then obtain an MRI scan of the head to exclude structural brainstem lesions such as Chiari malformation or brainstem tumor. Treatment of the structural brainstem lesion (eg, suboccipital decompression for Chiari malformation type 1) may improve RBD symptoms as well. In other instances, when appropriate, the patient might need to be evaluated by a developmental pediatrician to exclude an autism spectrum disorder, or a medical geneticist to diagnose Smith Magenis syndrome.

RSWA by itself does not need intervention, as it is only a polygraphic finding. It is important to ensure, however, that the patient with RSWA has not manifested overt RBD at other times previously. If the precipitating pharmacologic agent can be safely stopped or lowered in dose, this should be considered. With regard to pharmacologic therapy, agents such as clonazepam, 0.25 to 0.5 mg at bedtime, or melatonin, 1 to 3 mg at bedtime, can be considered. The length of time for which drug treatment needs to be continued is not known.

Finally, the safety of the child must be taken into consideration. As it is possible for the child to get out of bed with an RBD episode, this should be discussed with the child's caretakers, and appropriate measures should be employed to ensure the child's safety.

FUTURE DIRECTIONS

It would be helpful to develop a consensus among experts about whether the transitional sleep of the premature infant is analogous to RSWA.

There is a certain element of subjectivity involved on scoring augmented chin and leg electromyographic activity during REM sleep. Refinement in automated signal analysis techniques may facilitate diagnosis.

In both adults and children with RBD, the emphasis has been on describing the clinical features, neurologic or psychiatric comorbidities, and the predictive value in adults as possible biomarkers for a synucleinopathy. Surprisingly, there have been no studies on the mechanisms involved in terminating the RBD event. Should not the violent flailing of limbs during an RBD event trigger an immediate awakening that would then effectively terminate the event? Instead, the RBD events continue for 0.5 to 2 minutes. Is RBD a consequence of decreased ability to awaken from REM sleep, especially in those with hypocretin deficiency?

It is hoped that there will be increased interest in the study of childhood-onset RBD in the near future.

REFERENCES

1. Schenck CH, Bundlie SR, Patterson AL, et al. Rapid eye movement behavior disorder: a treatable parasomnia affecting older adults. JAMA 1987;257: 1786–9.
2. Stores G. Rapid eye movement sleep behavior disorder in children and adolescents. Dev Med Child Neurol 2008;50:728–32.
3. Navelet Y, Benoit O, Bouard G. Nocturnal sleep organization during the first months of life. Electroencephalogr Clin Neurophysiol 1982;54:71–8.
4. Partinen M, Hublin C. Epidemiology of sleep disorders. In: Kryger MH, Roth T, Dement WC, editors. Principles and practice of sleep disorders. Philadelphia: WB Saunders; 2000. p. 558–79.
5. American Academy of Sleep Medicine. The AASM manual for the scoring of sleep and associated events 2007. p. 41–3.
6. Boeve BF, Silber MH, Saper CB, et al. Pathophysiology of REM sleep behaviour disorder and elevance to neurodegenerative disease. Brain 2007; 130:2770–88.
7. Zangini S, Calandra-Buonaura G, Grimaldi D, et al. REM behavior disorder and neurodegenerative diseases. Sleep Med 2011;12:554–8.
8. Nightingale S, Orgill JC, Ebrahim IO, et al. The association between narcolepsy and REM behavior disorder (RBD). Sleep Med 2005;6:253–8.
9. Cipolli C, Francceschini C, Mattarozzi K, et al. Overnight distribution and motor characteristics of REM sleep behavior disorder episodes in patients with narcolepsy-cataplexy. Sleep Med 2011;12: 635–40.

10. Lloyd R, Tippmann-Peikert M, Slocumb N, et al. Characteristics of REM sleep behavior disorder in childhood. J Clin Sleep Med 2012;8(2):127–31.

11. Rye DB, Johnston LH, Watts RL, et al. Juvenile Parkinson's disease with REM sleep behavior disorder, sleepiness, and daytime REM onset. Neurology 1999;53:1868–70.

12. Henriques-Filho PS, Sergio PA, Pratesi R. Sleep apnea and REM sleep behavior disorder in patients with Chiari malformations. Arq Neuropsiquiatr 2008; 66:344–9.

13. Thirumalai SS, Shubin RA, Robinson R. Rapid eye movement sleep behavior disorder in children with autism. J Child Neurol 2002;17:173–8.

14. Sheldon SH, Jacobsen J. REM-sleep motor disorder in children. J Child Neurol 1998;13:257–60.

15. Nevsimalova S, Prihodova I, Kemlink D, et al. REM sleep behavior disorder (RBD) can be one of the first symptoms of childhood narcolepsy. Sleep Med 2007;8:784–6.

16. Trajanovic NN, Volch I, Shapiro CM, et al. REM sleep behavior disorder in a child with Tourette syndrome. Can J Neurol Sci 2004;31:572–5.

17. Teman PT, Tippmann-Peikert M, Silber MH, et al. Idiopathic rapid eye movement disorder: associations with antidepressants psychiatric diagnoses, and other factors in relation to age of onset. Sleep Med 2009;10:60–5.

18. Mahowald MW, Schenck CH. Dissociated states of wakefulness and sleep. Neurology 1992;42(7 suppl 6):44–51.

19. Schenck CH, Hurwitz TD, Mahowald MW. Normal and abnormal REM sleep regulation: REM sleep behavior disorder: an update on a series of 96 patients and a review of the world literature. J Sleep Res 1993;2:224–31.

20. Maski KP, Jeste SS, Spence SJ. Common neurological co-morbidities in autism spectrum disorders. Curr Opin Pediatr 2011;23:609–15.

21. Gropman AL, Duncan WC, Smith AC. Neurological and developmental features of the Smith Magenis syndrome (del 17 p11.2). Pediatr Neurol 2006;34: 337–50.

22. McNaught KS, Mink JW. Advances in understanding and treatment of Tourette syndrome. Nat Rev Neurol 2011;7:667–76.

Sleep-Related Breathing Disorder, Cognitive Functioning, and Behavioral-Psychiatric Syndromes in Children

Louise M. O'Brien, PhD, MS[a,b],*

KEYWORDS

- Sleep-disordered breathing • Behavioral outcome • Psychiatric outcomes • Cognitive outcomes

KEY POINTS

- Childhood sleep-disordered breathing (SDB) is robustly associated with behavioral disturbances such as hyperactivity, inattention, and aggression.
- Many studies find that cognitive problems and psychiatric disorders are more common in children with SDB than in those without.
- Dysfunction of the prefrontal cortex has been proposed as a mechanism linking sleep disruption to behavioral and cognitive problems.
- Nonetheless, the majority of children with SDB remain undiagnosed.

INTRODUCTION

There is a wealth of literature describing the relationships between sleep-disordered breathing (SDB), behavior, and cognition in children. Although these relationships were first recognized in the 1800s, it is only in recent decades that there has been a focus on the underlying pathophysiology, consequences, and treatment. This article summarizes current neurobehavioral and psychiatric manifestations of pediatric SDB.

PREVALENCE AND RISK FACTORS

SDB is a spectrum of breathing disturbances ranging from habitual snoring through to obstructive sleep apnea with associated sleep fragmentation and alterations in ventilation. Definitions of SDB vary, thus hampering accurate prevalence data, but a recent review of the epidemiology of pediatric SDB reported that "always snoring" occurs in 1.5% to 6.0% of children, with various constellations of SDB symptoms reported by questionnaire to occur in 4% to 20% of children.[1,2] Objective evidence of SDB from polysomnography, using various criteria, occurs in approximately 1% to 4% of children.[2]

The major risk factors for pediatric SDB are adenotonsillar hypertrophy and obesity. Symptoms of SDB have been reported in infancy,[3] although the majority of studies focus on elementary and middle school children. Although there does not seem to be a clear age-related pattern for SDB, young children are believed to be at greatest risk possibly owing to adenotonsillar tissue being largest relative to airway size. However, this belief has recently been questioned, because in normal children the growth of adenotonsillar tissue may

[a] Department of Neurology, Sleep Disorders Center, C736 Med Inn Building, Ann Arbor, MI 48109-5845, USA;
[b] Department of Oral & Maxillofacial Surgery, University of Michigan, 1500 East Medical Center Drive, Ann Arbor, MI 48109, USA
* Department of Neurology, Sleep Disorders Center, C736 Med Inn Building, Ann Arbor, MI 48109-5845.
E-mail address: louiseo@med.umich.edu

Sleep Med Clin 10 (2015) 169–179
http://dx.doi.org/10.1016/j.jsmc.2015.02.005
1556-407X/15/$ – see front matter © 2015 Elsevier Inc. All rights reserved.

actually be proportionate to airway growth, suggesting that any deviation from this trajectory would be abnormal.[4] Children with enlarged tonsils and adenoids may have increased upper airway collapsibility.[5] Several studies suggest that SDB may be more frequent in children of African-American race compared with Caucasians[6,7] and that boys may be at higher risk of SDB than girls,[8–10] especially in studies that included teenagers,[11] where pubertal hormonal changes likely contribute to the gender differences observed in adults. In addition, children with craniofacial anomalies and those with disorders affecting upper airway patency are at higher risk of SDB. Risk factors for SDB can include prenatal and perinatal complications, but such factors seem to become insignificant when controlling for socioeconomic status and race.[12]

CONSEQUENCES OF SLEEP-DISORDERED BREATHING

There is now a wealth of literature showing strong and significant associations between habitual snoring and/or objective measures of SDB with a range of neurobehavioral, cognitive, and psychiatric problems. Such consequences are likely related to interactions between the episodic hypoxemia and sleep fragmentation that characterize SDB. These outcomes have shown to be at least partially reversible after treatment for SDB, suggestive of a causal relationship. A summary of the relationships between SDB and behavioral, cognitive, and psychiatric outcomes is provided in this article.

BEHAVIORAL OUTCOMES

Behavioral problems demonstrate the most robust association with pediatric SDB, particularly hyperactive and inattentive behaviors. Furthermore, there is evidence suggestive of a role for SDB in conduct problems and aggressive behaviors. In the 1970s, Guilleminault and co-workers[13,14] reported on behavioral problems associated with SDB and since then this has remained a topic of considerable interest.

Hyperactivity

Hyperactivity has been reported in both children with habitual snoring,[15–23] as well as those in whom SDB was formally diagnosed by polysomnography.[24–31] Despite differences in definition of snoring or polysomnography-confirmed SDB, many studies support the relationship between snoring/SDB and hyperactive behaviors even when hyperactivity is measured with a range of

parent-report tools, including the Conners' Parent Rating Scales,[23–25,27] the Child Behavior Checklist,[24,26,29–31] or the Behavioral Assessment Scale for Children.[28,32] Only a small number of studies have failed to find associations with SDB and hyperactive behaviors.[33–35] The vast majority of published studies report cross-sectional findings that, although important, provide no information on the direction of the proposed relationships. More recently, some evidence in support of the hypothesis that SDB may play a causal role in hyperactive behaviors comes from a 4-year, prospective study in Michigan.[36] In this study, snoring and symptoms of SDB were strong risk factors for the future development or exacerbation of hyperactive behaviors, with habitual snoring at baseline increasing the risk for hyperactivity at follow-up by more than 4-fold. Findings were particularly strong in boys. Results were independent of hyperactivity at baseline and stimulant use as well as SDB symptoms at follow-up. This suggests that damage done 4 years earlier may have been visible as a hyperactive phenotype only years later, and alludes to the belief that there may be a "window of vulnerability" in developing humans.

Inattention

Attention is a critical behavior arising from brain mechanisms and is required for optimum learning. It describes a set of cognitive processes that can optimize the detection and discrimination of stimuli, as well as stimulus processing. Attention can be categorized as sustained, selective, and divided attention, thus representing a cluster of variables, each of which contribute to learning and memory. Inattentive behaviors identified by parental report have been observed in children with habitual snoring[15,17,23,37] and polysomnography-defined SDB,[28–30,32–34] although this finding is not as robust as the associations with hyperactivity. Different categories of attention, for example selective and sustained attention, can also be measured using objective assessments, such as auditory or visual continuous performance tests (CPT) and therefore may provide more robust assessment than parental report.

In a small study of 13 children who snored, in the absence of objective SDB, and 13 controls, Kennedy and colleagues[38] found that both selective and sustained attention measured objectively using the auditory CPT were found to be impaired by habitual snoring. Galland and colleagues[39] found that, in comparison with a normal population, children with objectively confirmed SDB, compared with those without, had significantly higher scores on a visual CPT for inattention and impulsivity albeit within the average range of a normal nonclinical score. Impaired auditory and visual attention has also been reported in children with objectively confirmed SDB compared with standardized norms.[40] Despite these findings, some studies fail to observe differences in visual attention.[28,41] Emancipator and associates[42] proposed that the CPT may either not be sufficiently sensitive in children who are not obviously sleepy or, possibly, with the increase in time children now spend playing video games, such CPT tools may be less discriminating.

Aggressive Behaviors

Aggressive and bullying behaviors are commonly observed among children, and estimates suggest that up to 25% of children in elementary schools are affected,[43] with a higher prevalence in boys.[44] Such behaviors present a major challenge not only for schools but also for society; aggressive children are at high risk for future psychiatric symptoms, violence, substance abuse, and criminality[45] and the victims of bullying also suffer. Although causes of aggressive behaviors are complex and include social, biological, and cultural factors, there is emerging evidence that sleep problems may play a role. In a large, population-based study of more than 3000 children who were 5 years old, those with symptoms of SDB were twice as likely to have parentally reported aggressive behaviors,[20] which is similar to the findings of Chervin and colleagues,[46] who also adjusted for comorbid hyperactivity and stimulant use.

In children with objectively confirmed SDB, aggressive behaviors are also more frequent than in children without SDB,[33] even when SDB is mild.[29] A recent study in an urban public school district, the first study specifically designed to investigate sleep problems in young children with aggressive behaviors,[47] showed that SDB was twice as common in children with aggression as compared with children without. However, sleepiness rather than a symptom more specific to SDB, such as snoring, seemed to drive the association between SDB risk and aggressive behaviors. Of note, short sleep duration, which perhaps may partially explain sleepiness, and sleep difficulties have been found to be associated with aggressive behaviors in young children[48,49] and with suicidal ideation in adolescents.[50]

Teacher Report of Behavior

There are conflicting findings on the association between SDB and behavior, depending on whether behavioral reports are by provided by parents or teachers. The literature regarding teacher reports is small compared with parental reports. Ali and colleagues[21] found that hyperactive and inattentive behavior scores were all increased in children with habitual snoring on both parent and teacher reports using Conners Rating Scales, whereas aggressive behaviors were only elevated by parent report. Arman and colleagues[17] found that, compared with their nonsnoring peers, children who snore habitually were more likely to have hyperactivity on the Conners Rating Scale by parental report, but not by teacher report. Studies using the Behavior Assessment System for Children (BASC) have found increases in hyperactivity and externalizing behaviors from parental report, but only increased externalizing behaviors in the teacher reports.[28] Recently, Beebe and colleagues[32] reported on children aged 10 to 17 years with varying severity of SDB. Using the BASC, parent reports of hyperactivity, attention, and aggression were all increased in children with SDB compared with children with no SDB, but the teacher reports were limited to differences in attention only. In a recent study from our group,[47] teacher-reported bullying behaviors did not show associations with symptoms of SDB, although parent reports did. The limited number of studies that have collected teacher reports, the different tools used, and the sample sizes involved make it difficult to reach conclusions regarding classroom behavior. However, despite the inconsistencies, the teacher report studies published to date seem to support a role for SDB in at least some areas of behavioral regulation.

COGNITIVE OUTCOMES

Cognition is a mental act or process by which knowledge is acquired, including awareness, perception, intuition, and reasoning. Because one of the fundamental roles of sleep is believed to be in learning, memory consolidation, and brain plasticity,[51] sleep disruption has the potential to impair cognition during wake. Indeed several studies, but not all,[52] find differences in cognition of children with and without SDB. The vast majority of studies in this area are from a limited age range, often elementary school age, thus limiting the conclusions that can be drawn.

The term 'cognition' is often used interchangeably with 'intelligence.' However, cognitive processes generally show an age-dependent performance increase, whereas intelligence typically refers to developmental differences between individuals.[53] In addition, cognitive processes can be influenced by intelligence. Lower order cognitive processes, which include perceptual motor learning, visual short-term memory, and selective attention, can be measured by tasks such as reaction times or problem solving. Intelligence, on the other hand, is indirectly inferred, typically via psychometric testing. A detailed discussion of the associations between sleep, cognition, and intelligence is beyond the scope of this article, but can be found in another recent article.[54]

Intelligence

Several studies have investigated the intelligence quotient (IQ) in children with SDB, although the findings are not consistent. Many studies report lower IQ scores in children with SDB compared with controls, although these scores are typically still within the normal range.[15,34,35,38,41,55–60] Kohler and colleagues[58] studied a group of snoring children awaiting adenotonsillectomy and found that, compared with healthy nonsnoring children, the snoring children had a 10-point reduction in IQ. Several studies have failed to find overall differences in full-scale IQ,[26,52,61,62] but some found lower scores for verbal IQ (language skills) in children with SDB.[26,61]

Notably, emerging data demonstrate score differences from standardized vocabulary tests—a measure of IQ—in children with and without SDB is equivalent to the impact of lead exposure.[63] These authors pointed out that vocabulary tests are the single best predictor of general cognitive functioning and are a strong predictor of academic success. Thus, SDB-related impairments may carry great clinical significance for future career achievements. Although ability to stay on task and pay attention in class may underlie learning ability, biological contributors including socioeconomic status, genetics, and obesity also play a role in cognitive outcomes.[32,64,65]

Memory

Differences in memory have been found in children with SDB, although the results are inconsistent, with several studies failing to find evidence for memory impairment.[15,34,66] In 1 study, memory was found to be impaired in children with SDB with a dose–response effect,[67] although in general most studies that find differences in memory do not find a dose response.[35,38,68] Inconsistencies in memory findings are likely related to the type of memory measured (such as verbal memory or working memory). In addition, many reports provide only a cumulative memory score rather than address specific processes involved in memory acquisition.

In a recent study,[68] 54 children with varying degrees of SDB and 17 controls completed a pictorial memory task and had their recall assessed both immediately and the next day. Memory recall on both occasions was impaired in children with SDB and the latter children also exhibited declines in recall performance that were absent in controls, suggesting that those with SDB require more time and additional learning opportunities to reach immediate and longer term recall performance. Furthermore, it has been suggested that children with SDB may have slower information processing and/or secondary memory problems and that inefficient encoding may account for the primary deficit.[69] This is supportive of data from an investigation of event-related potentials, which found no performance deficits on standard measures of attention and memory, but did find changes in basic perceptual processes that provide a foundation for the development of higher order functions.[70] Additional research is clearly required to understand the SDB-related impact on memory processes in children.

Academic Performance

Academic performance can be assessed by various means including mathematical abilities, spelling, reading, writing, and overall school grades. Studies have shown that symptoms of SDB in young children is associated with lower grades in mathematics, spelling, reading, and science,[37,71,72] even when intermittent hypoxemia is absent.[73] In first grade children, a 6- to 9-fold increase in gas exchange abnormalities was found in those with poor performance.[74] The presence of hypoxemia may affect the threshold of respiratory events associated with performance deficits; the threshold for respiratory disturbances associated with learning problems may be lower in the presence of hypoxemia.[75] Children with SDB have been found to perform lower than controls on a phonological processing test,[34,76] which measures phonological awareness, a skill that is critical for learning to read. However, not all studies find an association with SDB and academic achievement, particularly when other confounders such as socioeconomic status and preterm birth are accounted for.[35,42,77,78]

Interestingly, symptoms of SDB in early childhood have been associated with future risk for poor performance in middle school,[79] again suggesting that there may be a window of vulnerability whereby an insult at a key developmental time period may manifest phenotypically later on. A recent carefully matched study found a complex verbal skill profile in children with SDB.[80] Preschool children with SDB had difficulties in processing information with increasing linguistic complexity whereas the school-aged children had reduced vocabulary ability/knowledge. The authors postulated that their findings may support a longitudinal, adverse effect of SDB. Notably, the vast majority of current literature does not include adolescents, a developmental stage where challenges differ considerably from young children and where SDB-associated behavioral difficulties may result in significant impairment in school performance at a critical time for future success.[32] In addition to verbal problems, poor academic achievement may also be affected by inattention difficulties owing to the complex brain associations involved. Measurement of school performance is inherently difficult, and the role of SDB difficult to tease out, because it really represents a number of factors, which include age, socioeconomic status, home environment, genetics, behavior, and cognition.[32]

Executive Functions and Higher Cognitive Reasoning

Executive function encompasses cognitive processes, including memory, planning, problem solving, verbal reasoning, inhibition, mental flexibility, and multitasking, that are crucial for normal psychological and social development. Executive function is complex and it is difficult to isolate certain executive functions from other cognitive abilities; nonetheless, executive dysfunction has been found in school-age children with SDB compared with controls.[26,28,40,56] Even snoring preschool children have substantially lower performance on executive function dimensions, such as inhibition, working memory, and planning.[81] These findings underscore the need to identify SDB risk in young children. The importance of executive dysfunction and the involvement of the prefrontal cortex in SDB was reviewed recently[82] and a model linking sleep disruption, hypoxemia, and disruption of the prefrontal cortex was proposed.

Psychiatric Outcomes

Psychiatric disorders affect a significant number of American youth. The National Comorbidity Survey, a large nationally representative study of more than 10,000 adolescents aged 13 to 18 years estimated that the lifetime prevalence of having any one of a number of psychiatric disorders, including attention deficit hyperactivity disorder (ADHD), depressive disorder, anxiety disorder, conduct disorder, phobias, and drug/alcohol abuse is 49.5.[83] The lifetime prevalence for ADHD was reported as 4.2 in females and 13.0 in males, with that for conduct disorder being 5.8 in females and 7.9 in males, and depression being 15.9 in females and 7.7 in males. Although there is a body of

literature demonstrating associations between sleep problems and psychiatric disorders in children and adolescents, most studies report data on sleep quality and sleep duration rather than SDB. Nonetheless, SDB has been associated with several psychiatric disorders, which are described herein.

Attention Deficit Hyperactivity Disorder

As mentioned, the most robust associations with childhood SDB are hyperactive and inattentive behaviors. Because these behaviors are also the major features of ADHD, the relationship between sleep and ADHD is the focus of much research. Children with ADHD demonstrate a high frequency of sleep problems, including behavioral sleep disorders as well as symptoms of SDB, with a parentally reported frequency up to 5 times greater than controls.[84] The association may be somewhat skewed in early studies because sleep disturbance was included as part of diagnostic criteria in the Diagnostic and Statistical Manual of Mental Disorders III (DSM-III), but not in later versions. Nonetheless, children with ADHD have been reported to snore than their peers,[22,85,86] with snoring possibly more common in those with the hyperactive/impulsive subtype of ADHD.[87] However, polysomnographic data are less clear in terms of an association between SDB and ADHD, and many studies fail to find a consistent relationship.

A significant limitation of many studies of SDB and ADHD is that few studies have included formal diagnoses of ADHD, but rather used symptoms consistent with ADHD risk.[27] A retrospective study of children with a diagnosis of ADHD who attended a sleep clinic found that only 7% of these children had objectively confirmed SDB, whereas 36% had periodic limb movement disorder,[88] supportive of findings suggesting that periodic limb movements may mediate the relationship between SDB and hyperactivity.[89] In one of a very few studies to utilize prospective psychiatric diagnoses, school-age children undergoing polysomnography before adenotonsillectomy found DSM-IV diagnoses of ADHD in almost one-third of children, yet one-half of these children did not fulfill criteria for a diagnosis of ADHD 1 year after adenotonsillectomy.[90] A recent systematic review[91] that retained only 3 studies that had used rigorous criteria for ADHD suggests that children with ADHD are indeed more likely to have SDB, albeit rather mild in severity.

Depression

In adults, SDB has been associated with depressive symptoms as well as DSM-IV depressive disorder.[92] Although the data in children are limited, several studies have shown that subscales of the Child Behavior Checklist and BASC show higher scores for anxious/depressive symptoms in children with SDB compared with those without.[15,93,94] However, there are also a number of studies that fail to find elevated scores on the same scales.[28,31,33,95] One of the few studies to investigate specifically depressive symptoms in children with SDB was designed to address the significant confounder of obesity.[96] This study of 85 children aged 8 to 12 years old, one-half of whom were obese, included children who were referred for evaluation of suspected SDB. Using the Children's Depression Inventory as well as overnight polysomnography, the authors found that depressive scores were significantly worse in both obese and nonobese children with habitual snoring compared with controls; of note the presence of obesity was not able to explain the differences observed, nor was the severity of SDB, suggesting that snoring is associated independently with depressive symptoms. Recent data in young children aged 3 to 6 years old has also found that snoring in these preschool children is associated with symptoms of anxiety and depression.[61] Given the known relationships between mood difficulties and later antisocial and aggressive behaviors, it is important to recognize mood problems early; if SDB plays a role in mood dysregulation, then early screening may be warranted.

Anxiety Disorders

Anxiety disorders are among the most prevalent childhood psychiatric disorders, affecting between 5% and 10% of children[97] and are among the most common disorders in adolescence.[98] Although there are numerous studies associating sleep difficulties with anxiety,[49,99–101] these studies focus mostly on sleep regulation such as insomnia and sleep behavior problems. Longitudinal studies have also shown associations between sleep problems in childhood and the development of anxiety, depression, and emotional dysregulation years later, but again are related to sleep difficulties other than SDB.[102,103]

Similar to the depression literature, data demonstrating preliminary associations between SDB and anxiety are taken mostly from studies designed to look at behavioral outcomes in children with SDB using tools such as the Conners, Child Behavior Checklist, or BASC. A few studies have reported differences in subscale scores for anxiety/depression,[15,19,29,61,104] although several others do not support these findings.[28,31,94] There is currently no clear evidence that SDB, as a specific sleep disorder, is related to anxiety disorders. There are,

however, a number of cross-sectional studies demonstrating an association between SDB and broad indices of internalizing symptoms.[29,61,66]

Conduct Disorder

In addition to the aggressive behaviors discussed, conduct and disruptive disorders are beginning to receive more attention in the SDB literature. These conditions pose a particular problem for schools, which often have local, state, and national programs to address this public health issue.[105] Although studies of SDB and conduct problems are more limited than those of hyperactivity and inattention, a few investigations have found associations between parentally reported symptoms of SDB and conduct problems.[46,47] Conduct disorder is known to be associated with a multitude of well-studied social and cultural foundations, although it is possible that SDB or other reasons for sleep disruption may contribute to some of the behaviors. In a study from Germany, elementary school children who were habitual snorers at 2 time points approximately 13 months apart, compared with nonsnorers and former snorers, were found to have higher risk for conduct problems.[18] Interestingly, a recent study showed that although polysomnographic variables did not predict disruptive behavior disorder, esophageal pressure monitoring did,[106] perhaps suggesting that current polysomnographic measures may not be sensitive enough in the prediction of outcomes. Given the high prevalence of conduct disorder and disruptive behaviors in schools and the long-lasting consequences for both perpetrators and victims, identification of modifiable biological contributors such as SDB should be a high priority.

The Role of the Prefrontal Cortex

Beebe and Gozal[82] eloquently proposed a model that provides a potential explanation as to how SDB may impact cognition and behavior. In this model the authors propose that the 2 major components of SDB, namely sleep fragmentation and hypoxemia, disrupt the restorative sleep processes by alterations of the cellular and biochemical pathways in specific brain regions. Such disruptions in the prefrontal cortex can lead to the executive dysfunction often observed in children with SDB as well as the cognitive and behavioral difficulties also reported. Dysfunction of the prefrontal cortex has also been proposed as a mechanism linking inadequate sleep to problems with emotional regulation and attention.[107] This raises the question of whether sleepiness, which is common in a range of sleep disorders including poor sleep hygiene, may mediate the daytime impairment. Even a reduction of 1 hour of sleep in young children is associated with worse cognitive performance and higher hyperactivity scores.[108] Of note, the prefrontal cortex is the main generator of slow electroencephalogram waveforms and slowing of the electroencephalogram, likely reflecting sleepiness, has been observed in children with behavioral difficulties.[109,110]

SUMMARY

Childhood SDB is associated strongly with a range of cognitive and behavioral disturbances, including some psychiatric diagnoses. Despite this, the majority of children with symptoms of SDB go unrecognized, even though simple screening could identify children in need of further evaluation. Definitive evidence showing that SDB causes cognitive and behavioral impairment has yet to emerge, although a randomized controlled trial evaluating neuropsychological and health outcomes of treatment for SDB in children is currently underway.[111]

REFERENCES

1. Freeman K, Bonuck K. Snoring, mouth-breathing, and apnea trajectories in a population-based cohort followed from infancy to 81 months: a cluster analysis. Int J Pediatr Otorhinolaryngol 2012; 76(1):122–30.
2. Lumeng JC, Chervin RD. Epidemiology of pediatric obstructive sleep apnea. Proc Am Thorac Soc 2008;5(2):242–52.
3. Montgomery-Downs HE, Gozal D. Snore-associated sleep fragmentation in infancy: mental development effects and contribution of secondhand cigarette smoke exposure. Pediatrics 2006;117(3): e496–502.
4. Arens R, Sin S, Willen S, et al. Rhino-sinus involvement in children with obstructive sleep apnea syndrome. Pediatr Pulmonol 2010;45(10):993–8.
5. Marcus CL, McColley SA, Carroll JL, et al. Upper airway collapsibility in children with obstructive sleep apnea syndrome. J Appl Physiol (1985) 1994;77(2):918–24.
6. Rosen CL, Larkin EK, Kirchner HL, et al. Prevalence and risk factors for sleep-disordered breathing in 8- to 11-year-old children: association with race and prematurity. J Pediatr 2003;142(4):383–9.
7. Redline S, Tishler PV, Schluchter M, et al. Risk factors for sleep-disordered breathing in children. Associations with obesity, race, and respiratory problems. Am J Respir Crit Care Med 1999; 159(5 Pt 1):1527–32.
8. Delasnerie-Laupretre N, Patois E, Valatx JL, et al. Sleep, snoring and smoking in high school students. J Sleep Res 1993;2(3):138–42.
9. Archbold KH, Pituch KJ, Panahi P, et al. Symptoms of sleep disturbances among children at two general pediatric clinics. J Pediatr 2002;140(1):97–102.
10. Owens JA, Spirito A, McGuinn M, et al. Sleep habits and sleep disturbance in elementary school-aged children. J Dev Behav Pediatr 2000;21(1):27–36.
11. Sanchez-Armengol A, Ruiz-Garcia A, Carmona-Bernal C, et al. Clinical and polygraphic evolution of sleep-related breathing disorders in adolescents. Eur Respir J 2008;32(4):1016–22.
12. Calhoun SL, Vgontzas AN, Mayes SD, et al. Prenatal and perinatal complications: is it the link between race and SES and childhood sleep disordered breathing? J Clin Sleep Med 2010;6(3):264–9.
13. Guilleminault C, Eldridge FL, Simmons FB, et al. Sleep apnea in eight children. Pediatrics 1976; 58(1):23–30.
14. Guilleminault C, Korobkin R, Winkle R. A review of 50 children with obstructive sleep apnea syndrome. Lung 1981;159(5):275–87.
15. O'Brien LM, Mervis CB, Holbrook CR, et al. Neurobehavioral implications of habitual snoring in children. Pediatrics 2004;114(1):44–9.
16. Brockmann PE, Urschitz MS, Schlaud M, et al. Primary snoring in school children: prevalence and neurocognitive impairments. Sleep Breath 2011; 16(1):23–9.
17. Arman AR, Ersu R, Save D, et al. Symptoms of inattention and hyperactivity in children with habitual snoring: evidence from a community-based study in Istanbul. Child Care Health Dev 2005;31(6):707–17.
18. Urschitz MS, Eitner S, Guenther A, et al. Habitual snoring, intermittent hypoxia, and impaired behavior in primary school children. Pediatrics 2004; 114(4):1041–8.
19. Fagnano M, van Wijngaarden E, Connolly HV, et al. Sleep-disordered breathing and behaviors of inner-city children with asthma. Pediatrics 2009;124(1): 218–25.
20. Gottlieb DJ, Vezina RM, Chase C, et al. Symptoms of sleep-disordered breathing in 5-year-old children are associated with sleepiness and problem behaviors. Pediatrics 2003;112(4):870–7.
21. Ali NJ, Pitson DJ, Stradling JR. Snoring, sleep disturbance, and behaviour in 4–5 year olds. Arch Dis Child 1993;68(3):360–6.
22. Chervin RD, Dillon JE, Bassetti C, et al. Symptoms of sleep disorders, inattention, and hyperactivity in children. Sleep 1997;20(12):1185–92.
23. Chervin RD, Archbold KH, Dillon JE, et al. Inattention, hyperactivity, and symptoms of sleep-disordered breathing. Pediatrics 2002;109(3):449–56.
24. Zhao Q, Sherrill DL, Goodwin JL, et al. Association between sleep disordered breathing and behavior in school-aged children: the Tucson children's assessment of sleep apnea study. Open Epidemiol J 2008;1:1–9.

25. Melendres MC, Lutz JM, Rubin ED, et al. Daytime sleepiness and hyperactivity in children with suspected sleep-disordered breathing. Pediatrics 2004;114(3):768–75.

26. Lewin DS, Rosen RC, England SJ, et al. Preliminary evidence of behavioral and cognitive sequelae of obstructive sleep apnea in children. Sleep Med 2002;3(1):5–13.

27. O'Brien LM, Holbrook CR, Mervis CB, et al. Sleep and neurobehavioral characteristics of 5- to 7-year-old children with parentally reported symptoms of attention-deficit/hyperactivity disorder. Pediatrics 2003;111(3):554–63.

28. Beebe DW, Wells CT, Jeffries J, et al. Neuropsychological effects of pediatric obstructive sleep apnea. J Int Neuropsychol Soc 2004;10(7):962–75.

29. Bourke RS, Anderson V, Yang JS, et al. Neurobehavioral function is impaired in children with all severities of sleep disordered breathing. Sleep Med 2011;12(3):222–9.

30. Ting H, Wong RH, Yang HJ, et al. Sleep-disordered breathing, behavior, and academic performance in Taiwan schoolchildren. Sleep Breath 2011;15(1):91–8.

31. Rosen CL, Storfer-Isser A, Taylor HG, et al. Increased behavioral morbidity in school-aged children with sleep-disordered breathing. Pediatrics 2004;114(6):1640–8.

32. Beebe DW, Ris MD, Kramer ME, et al. The association between sleep disordered breathing, academic grades, and cognitive and behavioral functioning among overweight subjects during middle to late childhood. Sleep 2010;33(11):1447–56.

33. Mulvaney SA, Goodwin JL, Morgan WJ, et al. Behavior problems associated with sleep disordered breathing in school-aged children–the Tucson children's assessment of sleep apnea study. J Pediatr Psychol 2006;31(3):322–30.

34. O'Brien LM, Mervis CB, Holbrook CR, et al. Neurobehavioral correlates of sleep-disordered breathing in children. J Sleep Res 2004;13(2):165–72.

35. Kaemingk KL, Pasvogel AE, Goodwin JL, et al. Learning in children and sleep disordered breathing: findings of the Tucson Children's Assessment of Sleep Apnea (tuCASA) prospective cohort study. J Int Neuropsychol Soc 2003;9(7):1016–26.

36. Chervin RD, Ruzicka DL, Archbold KH, et al. Snoring predicts hyperactivity four years later. Sleep 2005;28(7):885–90.

37. Kim JK, Lee JH, Lee SH, et al. School performance and behavior of Korean elementary school students with sleep-disordered breathing. Ann Otol Rhinol Laryngol 2011;120(4):268–72.

38. Kennedy JD, Blunden S, Hirte C, et al. Reduced neurocognition in children who snore. Pediatr Pulmonol 2004;37(4):330–7.

39. Galland BC, Dawes PJ, Tripp EG, et al. Changes in behavior and attentional capacity after adenotonsillectomy. Pediatr Res 2006;59(5):711–6.

40. Archbold KH, Giordani B, Ruzicka DL, et al. Cognitive executive dysfunction in children with mild sleep-disordered breathing. Biol Res Nurs 2004;5(3):168–76.

41. Gottlieb DJ, Chase C, Vezina RM, et al. Sleep-disordered breathing symptoms are associated with poorer cognitive function in 5-year-old children. J Pediatr 2004;145(4):458–64.

42. Emancipator JL, Storfer-Isser A, Taylor HG, et al. Variation of cognition and achievement with sleep-disordered breathing in full-term and preterm children. Arch Pediatr Adolesc Med 2006;160(2):203–10.

43. Nansel TR, Overpeck M, Pilla RS, et al. Bullying behaviors among US youth: prevalence and association with psychosocial adjustment. JAMA 2001;285(16):2094–100.

44. Boulton MJ, Underwood K. Bully/victim problems among middle school children. Br J Educ Psychol 1992;62(Pt 1):73–87.

45. Kumpulainen K, Rasanen E. Children involved in bullying at elementary school age: their psychiatric symptoms and deviance in adolescence. An epidemiological sample. Child Abuse Negl 2000;24(12):1567–77.

46. Chervin RD, Dillon JE, Archbold KH, et al. Conduct problems and symptoms of sleep disorders in children. J Am Acad Child Adolesc Psychiatry 2003;42(2):201–8.

47. O'Brien LM, Lucas NH, Felt BT, et al. Aggressive behavior, bullying, snoring, and sleepiness in schoolchildren. Sleep Med 2011;12(7):652–8.

48. Komada Y, Abe T, Okajima I, et al. Short sleep duration and irregular bedtime are associated with increased behavioral problems among Japanese preschool-age children. Tohoku J Exp Med 2011;224(2):127–36.

49. Ivanenko A, Crabtree VM, Obrien LM, et al. Sleep complaints and psychiatric symptoms in children evaluated at a pediatric mental health clinic. J Clin Sleep Med 2006;2(1):42–8.

50. Wong MM, Brower KJ, Zucker RA. Sleep problems, suicidal ideation, and self-harm behaviors in adolescence. J Psychiatr Res 2011;45(4):505–11.

51. Walker MP. The role of sleep in cognition and emotion. Ann N Y Acad Sci 2009;1156:168–97.

52. Calhoun SL, Mayes SD, Vgontzas AN, et al. No relationship between neurocognitive functioning and mild sleep disordered breathing in a community sample of children. J Clin Sleep Med 2009;5(3):228–34.

53. Anderson M. Marrying intelligence and cognition - a developmental view. New York: Cambridge University Press; 2005.

54. Geiger A, Achermann P, Jenni OG. Sleep, intelligence and cognition in a developmental context: differentiation between traits and state-dependent aspects. Prog Brain Res 2010;185:167–79.

55. Blunden S, Lushington K, Kennedy D, et al. Behavior and neurocognitive performance in children aged 5–10 years who snore compared to controls. J Clin Exp Neuropsychol 2000;22(5): 554–68.

56. Halbower AC, Degaonkar M, Barker PB, et al. Childhood obstructive sleep apnea associates with neuropsychological deficits and neuronal brain injury. PLoS Med 2006;3(8):e301.

57. Suratt PM, Peruggia M, D'Andrea L, et al. Cognitive function and behavior of children with adenotonsillar hypertrophy suspected of having obstructive sleep-disordered breathing. Pediatrics 2006; 118(3):e771–81.

58. Kohler MJ, Lushington K, van den Heuvel CJ, et al. Adenotonsillectomy and neurocognitive deficits in children with Sleep Disordered Breathing. PLoS One 2009;4(10):e7343.

59. Bourke R, Anderson V, Yang JS, et al. Cognitive and academic functions are impaired in children with all severities of sleep-disordered breathing. Sleep Med 2011;12(5):489–96.

60. Miano S, Paolino MC, Urbano A, et al. Neurocognitive assessment and sleep analysis in children with sleep-disordered breathing. Clin Neurophysiol 2011;122(2):311–9.

61. Aronen ET, Liukkonen K, Simola P, et al. Mood is associated with snoring in preschool-aged children. J Dev Behav Pediatr 2009;30(2):107–14.

62. Hill CM, Hogan AM, Onugha N, et al. Increased cerebral blood flow velocity in children with mild sleep-disordered breathing: a possible association with abnormal neuropsychological function. Pediatrics 2006;118(4):e1100–8.

63. Suratt PM, Barth JT, Diamond R, et al. Reduced time in bed and obstructive sleep-disordered breathing in children are associated with cognitive impairment. Pediatrics 2007;119(2):320–9.

64. Montgomery-Downs HE, Jones VF, Molfese VJ, et al. Snoring in preschoolers: associations with sleepiness, ethnicity, and learning. Clin Pediatr (Phila) 2003;42(8):719–26.

65. Spruyt K, Gozal D. A mediation model linking body weight, cognition, and sleep disordered breathing. Am J Respir Crit Care Med 2012; 185(2):199–205.

66. Blunden S, Lushington K, Lorenzen B, et al. Neuropsychological and psychosocial function in children with a history of snoring or behavioral sleep problems. J Pediatr 2005;146(6):780–6.

67. Rhodes SK, Shimoda KC, Waid LR, et al. Neurocognitive deficits in morbidly obese children with obstructive sleep apnea. J Pediatr 1995;127(5):741–4.

68. Kheirandish-Gozal L, De Jong MR, Spruyt K, et al. Obstructive sleep apnoea is associated with impaired pictorial memory task acquisition and retention in children. Eur Respir J 2010;36(1):164–9.

69. Spruyt K, Capdevila OS, Kheirandish-Gozal L, et al. Inefficient or insufficient encoding as potential primary deficit in neurodevelopmental performance among children with OSA. Dev Neuropsychol 2009;34(5):601–14.

70. Key AP, Molfese DL, O'Brien L, et al. Sleep-disordered breathing affects auditory processing in 5–7-year-old children: evidence from brain recordings. Dev Neuropsychol 2009;34(5):615–28.

71. Urschitz MS, Wolff J, Sokollik C, et al. Nocturnal arterial oxygen saturation and academic performance in a community sample of children. Pediatrics 2005;115(2):e204–9.

72. Ravid S, Afek I, Suraiya S, et al. Sleep disturbances are associated with reduced school achievements in first-grade pupils. Dev Neuropsychol 2009; 34(5):574–87.

73. Urschitz MS, Guenther A, Eggebrecht E, et al. Snoring, intermittent hypoxia and academic performance in primary school children. Am J Respir Crit Care Med 2003;168(4):464–8.

74. Gozal D. Sleep-disordered breathing and school performance in children. Pediatrics 1998;102(3 Pt 1): 616–20.

75. Goodwin JL, Kaemingk KL, Fregosi RF, et al. Clinical outcomes associated with sleep-disordered breathing in Caucasian and Hispanic children–the Tucson Children's Assessment of Sleep Apnea study (TuCASA). Sleep 2003;26(5):587–91.

76. Lundeborg I, McAllister A, Samuelsson C, et al. Phonological development in children with obstructive sleep-disordered breathing. Clin Linguist Phon 2009;23(10):751–61.

77. Mayes SD, Calhoun SL, Bixler EO, et al. Nonsignificance of sleep relative to IQ and neuropsychological scores in predicting academic achievement. J Dev Behav Pediatr 2008;29(3):206–12.

78. Chervin RD, Clarke DF, Huffman JL, et al. School performance, race, and other correlates of sleep-disordered breathing in children. Sleep Med 2003;4(1):21–7.

79. Gozal D, Pope DW Jr. Snoring during early childhood and academic performance at ages thirteen to fourteen years. Pediatrics 2001;107(6): 1394–9.

80. Honaker SM, Gozal D, Bennett J, et al. Sleep-disordered breathing and verbal skills in school-aged community children. Dev Neuropsychol 2009; 34(5):588–600.

81. Karpinski AC, Scullin MH, Montgomery-Downs HE. Risk for sleep-disordered breathing and executive function in preschoolers. Sleep Med 2008;9(4): 418–24.

82. Beebe DW, Gozal D. Obstructive sleep apnea and the prefrontal cortex: towards a comprehensive model linking nocturnal upper airway obstruction to daytime cognitive and behavioral deficits. J Sleep Res 2002;11(1):1–16.

83. Merikangas KR, He JP, Burstein M, et al. Lifetime prevalence of mental disorders in U.S. adolescents: results from the National Comorbidity Survey Replication–Adolescent Supplement (NCS-A). J Am Acad Child Adolesc Psychiatry 2010;49(10): 980–9.

84. Corkum P, Tannock R, Moldofsky H. Sleep disturbances in children with attention-deficit/hyperactivity disorder. J Am Acad Child Adolesc Psychiatry 1998;37(6):637–46.

85. Rodopman-Arman A, Perdahli-Fis N, Ekinci O, et al. Sleep habits, parasomnias and associated behaviors in school children with attention deficit hyperactivity disorder (ADHD). Turk J Pediatr 2011;53(4):397–403.

86. Gau SS, Chiang HL. Sleep problems and disorders among adolescents with persistent and subthreshold attention-deficit/hyperactivity disorders. Sleep 2009;32(5):671–9.

87. LeBourgeois MK, Avis K, Mixon M, et al. Snoring, sleep quality, and sleepiness across attention-deficit/hyperactivity disorder subtypes. Sleep 2004;27(3):520–5.

88. Crabtree VM, Ivanenko A, Gozal D. Clinical and parental assessment of sleep in children with attention-deficit/hyperactivity disorder referred to a pediatric sleep medicine center. Clin Pediatr (Phila) 2003;42(9):807–13.

89. Chervin RD, Archbold KH, Dillon JE, et al. Associations between symptoms of inattention, hyperactivity, restless legs, and periodic leg movements. Sleep 2002;25(2):213–8.

90. Chervin RD, Ruzicka DL, Giordani BJ, et al. Sleep-disordered breathing, behavior, and cognition in children before and after adenotonsillectomy. Pediatrics 2006;117(4):e769–78.

91. Cortese S, Konofal E, Yateman N, et al. Sleep and alertness in children with attention-deficit/hyperactivity disorder: a systematic review of the literature. Sleep 2006;29(4):504–11.

92. Ohayon MM. The effects of breathing-related sleep disorders on mood disturbances in the general population. J Clin Psychiatry 2003;64(10):1195–200 [quiz: 274–6].

93. Stein MA, Mendelsohn J, Obermeyer WH, et al. Sleep and behavior problems in school-aged children. Pediatrics 2001;107(4):E60.

94. Mitchell RB, Kelly J. Child behavior after adenotonsillectomy for obstructive sleep apnea syndrome. Laryngoscope 2005;115(11):2051–5.

95. Goldstein NA, Post JC, Rosenfeld RM, et al. Impact of tonsillectomy and adenoidectomy on child behavior. Arch Otolaryngol Head Neck Surg 2000;126(4):494–8.

96. Crabtree VM, Varni JW, Gozal D. Health-related quality of life and depressive symptoms in children with suspected sleep-disordered breathing. Sleep 2004;27(6):1131–8.

97. Costello EJ, Mustillo S, Erkanli A, et al. Prevalence and development of psychiatric disorders in childhood and adolescence. Arch Gen Psychiatry 2003; 60(8):837–44.

98. Kessler RC, Avenevoli S, Costello EJ, et al. Prevalence, persistence, and sociodemographic correlates of DSM-IV disorders in the national comorbidity survey replication adolescent supplement. Arch Gen Psychiatry 2012;69(4):372–80.

99. Alfano CA, Zakem AH, Costa NM, et al. Sleep problems and their relation to cognitive factors, anxiety, and depressive symptoms in children and adolescents. Depress Anxiety 2009;26(6): 503–12.

100. Masi G, Millepiedi S, Mucci M, et al. Generalized anxiety disorder in referred children and adolescents. J Am Acad Child Adolesc Psychiatry 2004; 43(6):752–60.

101. Chase RM, Pincus DB. Sleep-related problems in children and adolescents with anxiety disorders. Behav Sleep Med 2011;9(4):224–36.

102. Johnson EO, Chilcoat HD, Breslau N. Trouble sleeping and anxiety/depression in childhood. Psychiatry Res 2000;94(2):93–102.

103. Gregory AM, Rijsdijk FV, Dahl RE, et al. Associations between sleep problems, anxiety, and depression in twins at 8 years of age. Pediatrics 2006;118(3):1124–32.

104. Owens J, Spirito A, Marcotte A, et al. Neuropsychological and behavioral correlates of obstructive sleep apnea syndrome in children: a preliminary study. Sleep Breath 2000;4(2):67–78.

105. Hahn R, Fuqua-Whitley D, Wethington H, et al. Effectiveness of universal school-based programs to prevent violent and aggressive behavior: a systematic review. Am J Prev Med 2007;33(Suppl 2): S114–29.

106. Chervin RD, Ruzicka DL, Hoban TF, et al. Esophageal pressures, polysomnography, and neurobehavioral outcomes of adenotonsillectomy in children. Chest 2012;142(1):101–10.

107. Dahl RE. The impact of inadequate sleep on children's daytime cognitive function. Semin Pediatr Neurol 1996;3(1):44–50.

108. Touchette E, Petit D, Seguin JR, et al. Associations between sleep duration patterns and behavioral/cognitive functioning at school entry. Sleep 2007; 30(9):1213–9.

109. Forssman H, Frey TS. Electroencephalograms of boys with behavior disorders. Acta Psychiatr Neurol Scand 1953;28(1):61–73.

110. Raine A, Venables PH, Williams M. Relationships between N1, P300, and contingent negative variation recorded at age 15 and criminal behavior at age 24. Psychophysiology 1990;27(5): 567–74.

111. Redline S, Amin R, Beebe D, et al. The Childhood Adenotonsillectomy Trial (CHAT): rationale, design, and challenges of a randomized controlled trial evaluating a standard surgical procedure in a pediatric population. Sleep 2011;34(11):1509–17.

Melatonin Treatment in Children with Developmental Disabilities

A.J. Schwichtenberg, PhD[a],*, Beth A. Malow, MD, MS[b]

KEYWORDS

- Melatonin • Sleep • Developmental disabilities • Autism • Smith–Magenis syndrome
- Angelman syndrome

KEY POINTS

- Melatonin is recommended commonly for children with developmental disabilities.
- Studies of melatonin efficacy in children with developmental disabilities document significantly shorter sleep onset latencies with melatonin treatment, which is best documented in children with autism spectrum disorders.
- Side effects of melatonin treatment were relatively uncommon and mild in nature.
- Melatonin to treat pediatric sleep disorders is not approved by the Food and Drug Administration, but studies provide promising evidence that melatonin could be effective in treating sleep-onset difficulties.

INTRODUCTION

Melatonin is the second most common medication recommended by clinicians for children with sleep disturbance (after antihistamines), with more than one-third recommending melatonin for children with developmental disabilities.[1] Despite its common use, relatively few clinical trials have documented the efficacy of melatonin in children with developmental disabilities. This review presents clinical trials, chart reviews, and case study reports (for less common developmental disabilities) of melatonin treatment. The intent of this review is to provide a succinct summary to help inform clinical and research practices for children with developmental disabilities. The developmental disabilities assessed include children with unspecified developmental delays or cognitive impairments and specific disorders/syndromes (eg, autism spectrum disorder, Smith-Magenis syndrome, Angleman's syndrome, fragile X syndrome, Down syndrome, and Rett syndrome).

PHARMACOLOGIC STUDIES
Diverse Developmental Disabilities

Until recently, most studies of melatonin efficacy have assessed groups of children with diverse developmental disabilities. These studies have included children with autism, cerebral palsy, 18q deletion syndrome, Angelman syndrome, ART-X syndrome, Bardet–Biedl syndrome, Down

Funding Sources: NIH/NIMH (R00 MH092431, PI: A.J. Schwichtenberg); NIH/NICHD (RO1 HD59253, Vanderbilt General Clinical Research Center), NIH/NCRR (M01 RR00095, PI: B.A. Malow).
Conflict of Interest: None to report.
[a] Department of Human Development and Family Studies, Department of Psychological Sciences, Department of Speech, Language, and Hearing Sciences, Purdue University, 1202 West State Street, West Lafayette, IN 47907-2055, USA; [b] Sleep Disorders Division, Department of Neurology, Vanderbilt University Medical Center, 1161 21st Avenue South, Room A-0116, Nashville, TN 37232-2551, USA
* Corresponding author. Department of Human Development and Family Studies, 1202 West State Street, West Lafayette, IN 47907-2055.
E-mail address: ajschwichtenberg@purdue.edu

syndrome, Prader–Willi syndrome, Sanfilippo syndrome, Saethre–Chotzen syndrome, 11q13 microdeletion, Leber amourosis, CHARGE syndrome, and unspecified intellectual deficits (ID). With the broad disability/syndrome composition of these studies, it can be difficult to draw conclusions for individual children or disorders/syndromes.[2] However, even with this challenge the published studies are relatively consistent. Short trials of melatonin (10 days–4 weeks), consistently report significant decreases in sleep onset latency by about 20 to 30 minutes.[3–6] Longer trials (3–72 months) also endorse shorter sleep latency over time.[7,8]

Reports of total sleep duration are less consistent, with about one-half of the studies of children with ID (stemming from various disorders/syndromes) reporting increases in sleep duration with melatonin treatment and one-half reporting no difference when compared with placebo (**Table 1**). Two studies—by Braam and colleagues[3] and De Leersnyder and colleagues[9]—reported a decrease in night awakenings, but 3 other studies of children with ID did not report a significant reduction in night awakenings with melatonin treatment.[6,7,10] Unlike early reports of melatonin use[11] and studies of specific disorders/syndromes, only one of the reviewed studies of children with ID reported melatonin-related side effects (daytime somnolence and naps).

Altered endogenous melatonin profiles have been documented in individuals with Down syndrome, Prader–Willi syndrome, and Sanfilippo syndrome.[12–15] However, for these conditions, we found minimal information on the efficacy or safety of melatonin treatment in children. In studies of diverse developmental disabilities, individuals with these syndromes were included, but syndrome-specific findings were not reported. Trials focusing on groups of children with these syndromes are needed to evaluate not only melatonin treatment efficacy, but also possible differences in how melatonin may be metabolized within these syndromes.

Autism Spectrum Disorder and Associated Genetic Conditions

Several studies have assessed the efficacy of melatonin in treating sleep disturbance in children with autism spectrum disorder (ASD) and associated genetic conditions (fragile X syndrome, tuberous sclerosis). Although the dose, duration, and elements of sleep affected by melatonin vary considerably across studies, the cumulative findings provide support for melatonin treatment.

The review presented herein is not an exhaustive list of ASD and melatonin studies. It focuses on the most recent studies and randomized, placebo-controlled trials. The reader is directed to recent reviews of melatonin in ASD, which have highlighted some of the limitations of prior studies (which are also applicable to studies of melatonin in other developmental disabilities).[16–18] These include (1) small sample size, (2) participants not limited to those with autism, (3) outcome measures of sleep are subjective (use of diaries rather than actigraphy, videosomnography, or polysomnography), (4) screening for medical comorbidities that can contribute to insomnia was not commonly done, (5) lack of parent- or child-directed sleep education, (6) assessment of effect on daytime behavior and family functioning was not performed, and (7) predictors of response (eg, endogenous melatonin, age, IQ) were not assessed. These reviews concluded that, although melatonin shows promise, large, randomized trials are needed to establish its efficacy.

In a chart review study of 107 children with ASD, Andersen and colleagues[19] reported that 85% of children who were treated with melatonin (0.75–6 mg) reported improvements in sleep. Several smaller retrospective studies also report improvements in sleep (to varying degrees). For example, in Gupta and Hutchins' study[20] of 9 children with autistic disorder, melatonin treatment (2.5–5 mg) was associated with shorter sleep onset latencies and longer sleep durations for about half of the children. In open-label trials, Paavonen and colleagues,[21] Giannotti and colleagues,[22] and Malow and colleagues[23] also reported decreases in sleep onset latency. Garstang and Wallis[24] completed a randomized, double-blind, crossover trial with 11 children with ASD, revealing shorter sleep onset latency times, fewer night awakenings, and longer total sleep durations with melatonin treatment (5 mg). Similarly, Wirojanan and colleagues[25] reported shorter sleep onset latencies, longer nighttime sleep durations, and earlier sleep onset times with melatonin treatment (3 mg) in a randomized, double-blind, crossover trial of 11 children with ASD and/or fragile X syndrome. In a slightly larger randomized, double-blind, controlled trial of 17 children with ASD, Wright and associates[26] reported shorter sleep onset latency and longer total sleep times with melatonin treatment ($\leq$10 mg). In the largest randomized placebo-controlled trial to date, Cortesi and colleagues[27] studied134 children (69 of whom received controlled-release melatonin, 3 mg) and reported reduced sleep onset time and duration and increased sleep duration and efficiency. These improvements were reported for children who received cognitive–behavioral therapy and/or melatonin, but not for children in the placebo group.

A study of girls with Rett syndrome echoed the ASD studies and reported decreased sleep onset time and total sleep duration with melatonin treatment (2.5–7.5 mg).[28] Conversely, in a study of 5 children with tuberous sclerosis, a genetic condition associated with increased ASD risk, no significant sleep differences were noted in a 4-week randomized cross-over study of melatonin treatment.[29] Similarly, O'Callaghan and colleagues[30] did not report a decrease in sleep onset latency in their study of 7 individuals with tuberous sclerosis. However, they did report an increase in nighttime sleep duration. These studies highlight that ASD etiology may affect melatonin efficacy and etiology (when known) should be considered when assessing melatonin as a treatment option.

The most consistent finding across studies of children with ASD and associated genetic conditions is decreases in sleep onset latency. Findings regarding other elements of sleep are less consistent. For example, some studies report increased night awakenings and others report decreased night awakenings.[21,24] Although this inconsistency and others like it could stem from differences in dose, melatonin type (fast release or continuous release), administration time, duration of administration, and sleep measurement technique as well as individual differences in melatonin metabolism.

Melatonin's mechanism of influence in children with ASD is largely unknown. Although prior studies of nocturnal blood melatonin,[31] daytime blood melatonin,[32] and nocturnal melatonin metabolites[33] have suggested a melatonin deficiency in ASD, a recent study of endogenous melatonin profiles in 11 children with ASD responding to supplemental melatonin highlighted that pretreatment endogenous melatonin levels are neither low or delayed compared with normative values.[34] This indicates that the pathway of influence in ASD may not simply be low level melatonin replacement, but rather other melatonin effects (eg, hypnotic, phase shifting, or antianxiolytic).

Overall, studies of melatonin in children with ASD are promising and report relatively few side effects (ie, headaches, vomiting, upset stomach, dizziness, diarrhea, daytime sleepiness). Considering the relatively low rate(s) of side effects and the consistent findings regarding sleep onset latency, melatonin treatment for children with ASD who struggled with sleep onset is supported by the literature. Other types of sleep disturbances (eg, early morning awakenings, several nighttime awakenings, circadian rhythm shifts) may be treated with melatonin, but the research findings in these areas are less consistent.

Smith–Magenis Syndrome

Previous studies highlight circadian rhythm problems in some children with Smith–Magenis syndrome (SMS) reporting higher endogenous melatonin levels during the day than at night.[9,35] Several case studies report effectively treating circadian sleep disturbances using melatonin and β1-adrengic antagonists.[36–39] A research group from France carefully followed 9 children with SMS and reported a reversal of melatonin patterns with the treatment of β1-adrenergic antagonists during the day and melatonin before bedtime.[9] In total, these studies reflect the treatment of only 13 children. However, within a rare disorder such as SMS they present growing evidence that melatonin treatment (coupled with a β1-adrenergic antagonist) may help children with SMS who present with inverted or altered circadian patterns. Further support is provided in a series examining open-label use of prolonged-release melatonin in 88 children with neurodevelopmental disorders, 47 of whom had SMS, which documented improvements in parent-reported sleep latency, sleep duration, night awakenings, and sleep quality.[9]

Angelman Syndrome

We identified 2 small studies of children with Angelman syndrome. The first was an open-label trial in 13 children by Zhdanova and colleagues[40] wherein sleep duration increased from baseline levels with melatonin treatment (0.3 mg). However, Zhdanova and colleagues also reported lower overall activity levels (as indexed by an actigraph) which in and of itself may have affected the actigraph estimates of sleep. A second study by Braam and associates[41] was a randomized, double-blind, placebo-controlled study of 8 individuals with Angelman syndrome. This study reported several improvements in sleep with melatonin (2.5–5 mg), when compared with baseline and placebo, including shorter sleep onset latencies, earlier sleep onset time, fewer night awakenings, and longer sleep durations. Melatonin treatment for children with Angelman syndrome requires more research before conclusions regarding its efficacy and safety may be drawn but the current studies provide a positive backdrop for further research.

Table 1
Summary of melatonin efficacy studies for children with developmental disabilities

	Participants			Melatonin Treatment				Sleep Parameter						
Reference	Diagnosis	n	Age (y)	mg	Duration[a]	Side Effects[b]	Design	SO Latency	SO Time	Sleep Duration	Awakenings	Nights with Awakenings	Sleep Offset	Sleep Efficiency
Andersen et al,[19] 2008	ASD	107	2–18	.75–6	Varied	Sleepiness, enuresis	CR	—	—	—	—	—	—	—
Braam et al,[3] 2008	ID[c]	58	2–78	2.5–5	4 wk	None	R, DB, PC	↓	↓	↑	↓	NS	NS	—
Braam et al,[41] 2008	Angelman syndrome	8	4–20	2.5–5	4 wk	None	R, DB, PC	↓	↓	↑	NS	NS	NS	—
Camfield et al,[10] 1996	ID	6	3–13	.5–1	2 wk	None	DB, PC	—	—	NS	NS	NS	—	—
Coppola et al,[4] 2004	ID[d]	25	3–26	3–9	4 wk	None	DB, PC	↓	—	NS	NS	—	—	—
Cortesi et al,[27] 2012	ASD	134	4–10	3	12 wk	None	R, PC	↓	↓	↑	—	—	—	↑
De Leersnyder et al,[9] 2011	ID[e]	88	6–12	2–10	3–72 mo	Daytime somnolence or naps	OL	↓	—	↑	↓	—	↑	↑
Dodge and Wilson,[5] 2001	ID	20	1–12	5	2 wk	None	DB, PC	↓	—	NS	NS	—	—	—
Giannotti et al,[22] 2006	ASD	25	2–9	3–6	6 mo	None	OL	↓	↓	↑	↓	—	↑	—
Garstang and Wallis,[24] 2006	ASD	7	4–16	5	4 wk	None	R, DB, PC	↓	—	↑	—	—	—	—
Gringras et al,[8] 2012	ID	70	3–15	.5–12	12 wk	Melatonin = placebo	R, DB, PC	↓	—	↑	—	—	—	NS
Gupta and Hutchins,[20] 2005	ASD	9	2–11	2.5–5	1 wk–1 y	None	CR	↓	—	↑	—	—	—	—

Hancock et al,[29] 2005	Tuberous sclerosis	8	1–31	5–10	2 wk	None	R, DB, PC	NS	—	NS	NS	—	—	—
Malow et al,[23] 2012	ASD	24	3–10	1–6	15 wk	Loose stools	OL	↓	—	NS	—	—	—	NS
McArthur and Budden,[28] 1998	Rett syndrome	9	4–17	2.5–7.5	4 wk	Mood swings	DB, PC	↓	—	NS	NS	—	—	NS
O'Callaghan et al,[30] 1999	Tuberous sclerosis	7	2–28	5	2 wk	None	R, DB, PC	NS	—	↑	NS	—	—	—
Paavonen et al,[21] 2003	Asperger disorder	15	6–17	3	2 wk	Tiredness, headaches	OL	↓	—	NS	↑	—	—	NS
Wirojanan et al,[25] 2009	ASD, FXS	12	2–15	3	2 wk	None	R, DB, PC	↓	→	↑	NS	—	—	—
Wasdell et al,[6] 2008	ID	50	2–18	5	10–20 d, 3 mo	None	R, DB, PC, OL	↓	—	↑	NS	—	—	NS
Wright et al,[26] 2011	ASD	17	4–16	2–10	3 mo	Melatonin = placebo	R, DB, PC	↓	—	↑	NS	—	—	NS
Zhdanova et al,[40] 1999	Angelman syndrome	13	2–10	.3	1 wk	None	OL	—	—	↑	—	—	—	—

Abbreviations: ASD, autism spectrum disorder; CR, chart review; DB, double-blind; ID, intellectual deficits; FXS, fragile X syndrome; NS, no statically significant change with melatonin treatment; OL, open label; PC, placebo controlled; R, randomized; SO, sleep onset; —, not assessed in study; ↓, decreased (or was earlier) with melatonin treatment; ↑, increased (or was later) with melatonin treatment.

a Duration of melatonin treatment.
b Reported side effects.
c Autism, cerebral palsy, 18q deletion syndrome, Angelman syndrome, ART-X syndrome, Bardet–Biedl syndrome, Down syndrome, Prader–Willi syndrome, Sanfilippo syndrome.
d Angelman syndrome, Saethre–Chotzen syndrome, 11q13 microdeletion, Leber amourosis, CHARGE syndrome.
e Smith–Magenis syndrome, intellectual disability, encephalopathy, autism, Angleman syndrome, Rett syndrome, Bourneville syndrome, blindness.

SUMMARY/DISCUSSION

Studies of melatonin treatment for children with developmental disabilities provide mounting evidence of its efficacy and safety. The studies reviewed here and a recent meta-analysis by Braam and associates report beneficial effects with melatonin treatment with minimal side effects.[42] With the exception of tuberous sclerosis, every study reviewed (see **Table 1**) reported a significant decrease in sleep onset latency with melatonin treatment. Even with these promising reports it is important to note that melatonin is not approved by the US Food and Drug Administration; in fact, no drug (or supplement) is approved for use in pediatric insomnia. However, the off-label use of melatonin is common, especially in children with developmental disabilities.[1] Based on this review, melatonin is most effective in treating sleep onset difficulties and may be beneficial for other elements of sleep depending on child-specific factors. Additional studies, including large randomized trials, are needed to establish its efficacy and the variables that may influence treatment response.

REFERENCES

1. Owens J, Rosen C, Mindell J, et al. Use of pharmacotherapy for insomnia in child psychiatry practice: a National Survey. Sleep Med 2010;11(7): 692–700.
2. Guénolé F, Baleyte JM. Effects of melatonin should be studies separately in each neurodevelopmental disorder and with specific sleep diagnoses. Pediatr Neurol 2012;46:60–1.
3. Braam W, Didden R, Smits M, et al. Melatonin treatment in individuals with intellectual disability and chronic insomnia: a randomized placebo-controlled study. J Intellect Disabil Res 2008;52:256–64.
4. Coppola G, Iervolino G, Mastrosimone M, et al. Melatonin in wake- sleep disorders in children, adolescents, and young adults with mental retardation with or without epilepsy: a double-blind, cross-over, placebo-controlled trial. Brain Dev 2004;26:373–6.
5. Dodge N, Wilson AG. Melatonin for treatment of sleep disorders in children with developmental disabilities. J Child Neurol 2001;16:581–4.
6. Wasdell M, Jan J, Bomben M, et al. A randomized, placebo-controlled trail of controlled release melatonin treatment of delayed sleep phase syndrome and impaired sleep maintenance in children with neurodevelopmental disabilities. J Pineal Res 2008;4:57–64.
7. De Leersnyder H, de Blois M, Vekemans M, et al. β₁-adrenergic antagonists improve sleep and behavioural disturbances in a circadian disorder, Smith-Magenis syndrome. J Med Genet 2001;38: 586–90.
8. Gringras P, Gamble C, Jones AP, et al. Melatonin for sleep problems in children with neurodevelopmental disorders: randomised double masked placebo controlled trial. Br Med J 2012;345:e6664.
9. De Leersnyder H, Zisapel N, Laudon M. Prolonged-release melatonin for children with neurodevelopmental disorders. Pediatr Neurol 2011;45:23–6.
10. Camfield P, Gordon K, Dooley J, et al. Melatonin appears ineffective in children with intellectual deficits and fragmented sleep: six "N of 1" trials. J Child Neurol 1996;11:341–3.
11. Sheldon H. Pro-convulsant effects of oral melatonin in neurologically disabled children. Lancet 1998; 351:1254.
12. Butler M, Brandau D, Theodoro M, et al. Morning melatonin levels in Prader- Willi syndrome. Am J Med Genet 2009;149A:1809–13.
13. Guerroro J, Pozo D, Diaz-Rodriguez J, et al. Impairment of the melatonin rhythm in children with Sanfilippo syndrome. J Pineal Res 2006;40:192–3 [Letter to the Editor].
14. Tamarkin L, Abastillas P, Chen HC, et al. The daily profile of plasma melatonin in obese and Prader-Willi syndrome children. J Clin Endocrinol Metab 1982;55(3):491–5.
15. Uberos J, Romero J, Molina-Carballo A, et al. Melatonin and elimination of kynurenines in children with Down's syndrome. J Pediatr Endocrinol Metab 2010; 23(3):277–82.
16. Doyen C, Mighiu D, Kaye K, et al. Melatonin in children with autistic spectrum disorders: recent and practical data. Eur Child Adolesc Psychiatry 2011; 20:231–9.
17. Guénolé F, Godbout R, Nicolas A, et al. Melatonin for disordered sleep in individuals with autism spectrum disorders: systematic review and discussion. Sleep Med Rev 2011;15:379–87.
18. Rossignol D, Frye R. Melatonin in autism spectrum disorders: a systemic review and meta-analysis. Dev Med Child Neurol 2011;53(9):783–92.
19. Andersen MI, Kaczmarska J, McGrew GS, et al. Melatonin for insomnia in children with autism spectrum disorders. J Child Neurol 2008;23:482–5.
20. Gupta R, Hutchins J. Melatonin: a panacea for desperate parents? (Hype or truth). Arch Dis Child 2005;90:986–7.
21. Paavonen EJ, Nieminen-von Went T, Vanhala R, et al. Effectiveness of melatonin in the treatment of sleep disturbances in children with Asperger disorder. J Child Adolesc Psychopharmacol 2003;13:83–95.
22. Giannotti F, Cortesi F, Cerquiglini A, et al. An open-label study of controlled release melatonin in treatment of sleep disorders in children with autism. J Autism Dev Disord 2006;36:741–52.

23. Malow B, Adkins K, McGrew S, et al. Melatonin for sleep in children with autism: a controlled trail examining dose, tolerability, and outcomes. J Autism Dev Disord 2012;42:1729–37.

24. Garstang J, Wallis M. Randomized controlled of melatonin for children with autistic spectrum disorders and sleep problems. Child Care Health Dev 2006;32:585–9.

25. Wirojanan J, Jacquemont S, Siaz R, et al. The efficacy of melatonin for sleep problems in children with autism, fragile X syndrome or autism and fragile X syndrome. J Clin Sleep Med 2009;5(2):145–50.

26. Wright B, Sims D, Smart S, et al. Melatonin versus placebo in children with autism spectrum conditions and severe sleep problems not amenable to behavior management strategies: a randomized controlled crossover trial. J Autism Dev Disord 2011;41:175–84.

27. Cortesi F, Giannotti F, Sebastiani T, et al. Controlled-release melatonin, singly and combined with cognitive behavioural therapy, for persistent insomnia in children with autism spectrum disorders: a randomized placebo-controlled trial. J Sleep Res 2012;21:700–9.

28. McArthur AJ, Budden SS. Sleep dysfunction in Rett syndrome: a trial of exogenous melatonin treatment. Dev Med Child Neurol 1998;40:186–92.

29. Hancock E, O'Callaghan F, Osborne J. Effect of melatonin dosage on sleep disorder in tuberous sclerosis complex. J Child Neurol 2005;20:78–80.

30. O'Callaghan JF, Clarke AA, Hancoack E, et al. Use of melatonin to treat sleep disorders in tuberous sclerosis. Dev Med Child Neurol 1999;41:123–6.

31. Kulman G, Lissoni P, Rovelli F, et al. Evidence of pineal endocrine hypofunction in autistic children. Neuro Endocrinol Lett 2000;21:31–4.

32. Melke J, Goubran Botros H, Chaste P, et al. Abnormal melatonin synthesis in autism spectrum disorders. Mol Psychiatry 2008;13:90–8.

33. Tordjman S, Anderson GM, Pichard N, et al. Nocturnal excretion of 6-sulphatoxymelatonin in children and adolescents with autistic disorder. Biol Psychiatry 2005;57(2):134–8.

34. Goldman S, Adkins K, Wade Calcutt M, et al. Melatonin in children with autism spectrum disorders: endogenous and pharmacokinetic profiles in relation to sleep. J Autism Dev Disord 2014; 44:2525–35.

35. Potocki L, Glaze D, Tan D, et al. Circadian rhythm abnormalities of melatonin in Smith-Magenis syndrome. J Med Genet 2000;37:428–33.

36. Carpizo R, Martinez A, Mediavilla D, et al. Smith-Magenis syndrome: a case report of improved sleep after treatment with β_1-adrenergic antagonists and melatonin. J Pediatr 2006;149:409–11.

37. Chou I, Tsai F, Yu M, et al. Smith Magenis syndrome with bilateral vesicoureteral reflux: a case report. J Formos Med Assoc 2002;101:726–8.

38. Hou JW. Smith-Magenis syndrome: report of one case. Acta Paediatr Taiwan 2003;44:161–4.

39. Van Thillo A, Devriendt K, Willekens D. Sleep disturbances in Smith Magenis syndrome: treatment with melatonin and beta-adrenergic antagonists [abstract]. Tijdschr Psychiatr 2010;52(10):719–23.

40. Zhdanova I, Wurtman R, Wagstaff J. Effects of low dose melatonin on sleep in children with Angelman syndrome. J Pediatr Endocrinol Metab 1999;12:57–67.

41. Braam W, Didden R, Smits M, et al. Melatonin for chronic insomnia in Angelman syndrome: a randomized placebo-controlled trial. J Child Neurol 2008; 23:649–54.

42. Braam W, Smits M, Didden R, et al. Exogenous melatonin for sleep problems in individuals with intellectual disability: a meta-analysis. Dev Med Child Neurol 2009;51:340–9.

Printed and bound by CPI Group (UK) Ltd, Croydon, CR0 4YY

03/10/2024

01040366-0002